MILITANT LACTIVISM?

Fertility, Reproduction and Sexuality

GENERAL EDITORS:
David Parkin, Fellow of All Souls College, University of Oxford
Soraya Tremayne, Founding Director, Fertility and Reproduction Studies Group, and Research Associate, Institute of Social and Cultural Anthropology, University of Oxford
Marcia C. Inhorn, William K. Lanman, Jr. Professor of Anthropology and International Affairs, Yale University
Philip Kreager, Director, Fertility and Reproduction Studies Group, and Research Associate, Institute of Social and Cultural Anthropology and Institute of Human Sciences, University of Oxford

MILITANT LACTIVISM?
ATTACHMENT PARENTING AND INTENSIVE MOTHERHOOD IN THE UK AND FRANCE

Charlotte Faircloth

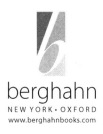

berghahn
NEW YORK · OXFORD
www.berghahnbooks.com

First published in 2013 by
Berghahn Books
www.BerghahnBooks.com

© 2013 Charlotte Faircloth

Library of Congress Cataloging-in-Publication Data

Faircloth, Charlotte.
 Militant lactivism : attachment parenting and intensive motherhood in the UK and France / Charlotte Faircloth.
  p. cm. — (Fertility, reproduction and sexuality ; . 24)
 Includes bibliographical references and index.
 ISBN 978-0-85745-758-5 (hardback : alk. paper) -- ISBN 978-0-85745-759-2 (institutional ebook)
  1. Breastfeeding—England. 2. Breastfeeding—France. 3. Infants—Nutrition—England. 4. Infants—Nutrition—France. 5. Parenting—Social aspects. I. Title.
 RJ216.F35 2013
 649′.330941—dc23

                                                              2012019036

British Library Cataloguing in Publication Data

A catalogue record for this book is available from the British Library.

Printed in the United States on acid-free paper

ISBN 978-0-85745-758-5 (hardback)
ISBN 978-0-85745-759-2 (institutional ebook)

CONTENTS

List of Illustrations

Figures

Tables

Epigraph

The anthropologist's role is not to question the facts of nature but to insist upon the interposition of a middle term between 'nature' and 'human behaviour'; his role is to analyse that term, to document local man-made doctorings of nature, and to insist that these doctorings should not be read off in any one culture as nature itself. Although it is a fact of nature that the child becomes a man, the way in which this transition is effected varies from one society to another, and no one of these particular cultural bridges should be regarded as the 'natural' path to maturity.

Ruth Benedict

ACKNOWLEDGEMENTS

First thanks go to the mothers who shared their experiences of breastfeeding with me: they taught me so much, both about being a mother and about being an anthropologist. I particularly want to thank the women in La Leche League who made my research possible. I know not all of them have been happy with my 'anthropological processing', but I do want to convey my warmest thanks for their welcoming, caring and reflexive approach to my project. I hope they will consider this a sensitive engagement with their accounts.

I am extremely grateful to the Foundation for the Sociology of Health and Illness and its award of the Mildred Blaxter Post-doctoral Fellowship, which has given me the opportunity to publish this research whilst based at the University of Kent. During my PhD studies in Cambridge, the Economic and Social Research Council, Pembroke College and the Ling Roth Fund provided generous funding that gave me the freedom to research and write, as well as attend numerous interesting events both in the UK and abroad.

I owe an intellectual debt to many people, as the text here will attest. In Cambridge, I am grateful to Françoise Barbira-Freedman, my PhD supervisor, who guided me through the research process with 'loving guidance', and to Marilyn Strathern and Yael Navaro-Yashin for their comments on my work. I am grateful to Barbara Bodenhorn, Stephen Hugh-Jones and Perveez Mody for their many years of support and encouragement. Members of the Centre for Family Research and the Centre for Gender Studies in Cambridge, particularly Martin Richards, Susan Golombok and Jude Browne, are also acknowledged here for bringing their interdisciplinary perspectives to bear on my research. In Kent, I am grateful to Ellie Lee, my postdoctoral mentor and director of the Centre for Parenting Culture Studies, who has taken an interest in my work from the very beginning and contextualised it as part of a growing body of work that explores the concept of parenting. Thanks too to Frank Furedi, Jennie Bristow and Jan Macvarish in particular for their input along the way. Further afield, I am grateful to Allison James for her astute reading of my work, to Elizabeth Murphy for her encouragement in thinking outside the anthropological discipline, to Linda Layne for mentoring me on a visiting scholarship to the US and to Diane Hoffman for her enthusiastic collaboration on several projects in the years since.

I was delighted that Berghahn agreed to publish this text as part of their *Fertility, Reproduction and Sexuality* series, and I thank both the publisher and the three editors of the series (Marcia Inhorn, David Parkin and Soraya Tremayne) for their support in this process. I am also grateful to the three readers of the first draft of this manuscript – their comments helped me shape it into what (I hope) is a more readable book overall.

Grateful thanks to the artist Heather Cushman-Dowdee for allowing me to reproduce her work here. The Cow Goddess's intervention, and the comments in the forum, really helped me to frame this research, as the text here will reflect. Thanks too to Best Beginnings for allowing me to reproduce a poster of theirs here.

Peers who have provided intellectual stimulation and friendship include Jonathan Beckman, Katie Dow, Zeynep Gürtin, Ann Kelly, Ofra Koffman, Virginia Langum, Nick Long, Nayanika Mathur, Ella McPherson, Laura Mentore, Annabel Pinker, Amy Pollard, Emilia Sanabria, Umut Yildirim and Naomi Wood. Thank you all. I am also grateful to members of the Cambridge Interdisciplinary Reproduction Forum for wonderful discussion and collaboration over the years.

Final thanks go to my family, who have supported the (what must seem endless) process of completing a book with patience and much love. Special thanks to Amol Rajan; you have been both intellectually demanding and kind, which is a rare but wonderful combination.

This book, however, could only ever be for one person – my mother.

I am grateful to the publishers concerned for the permission to use material that has appeared in the following:

Faircloth, C. 2011. '"It Feels Right in My Heart": Affect as Accountability in Narratives of Attachment', *Sociological Review* 59(2): 283–302.

Faircloth, C. 2010. 'What Science Says Is Best: Parenting Practices, Scientific Authority and Maternal Identity', *Sociological Research Online* (Special Section on 'Changing Parenting Culture') 15(4).

Faircloth, C. 2010. '"If They Want to Risk the Health and Well-Being of Their Child, That's Up to Them": Long-Term Breastfeeding, Risk and Maternal Identity', *Heath, Risk and Society* (Special Issue 'Child-Rearing in an Age of Risk') 12(4): 357–367.

Faircloth, C. 2009. "Culture Means Nothing to Me': Thoughts on Nature/Culture in Narratives of "Full-Term" Breastfeeding', *Cambridge Anthropology*, 28(2): 63–85.

INTRODUCTION

Starbucks, 14th arrondissement, Paris: I have arranged to meet a woman called Caroline. I am hoping she might be able to offer a few pointers on my proposed study of infant feeding practices, comparing rates of breastfeeding and formula feeding in London and Paris. She is a 'breastfeeding counsellor' with whom I have been put in touch by a woman in my language class, who described her as '*the* person you need to see in Paris – she knows everything there is to know about breastfeeding'. Naively, I do not approach the meeting as 'fieldwork'. Rather, I see Caroline as a potential gatekeeper (to the gatekeepers) to potential participants in my research.

A tall, slim, well-groomed woman walks into the café. She is talking to a child in school uniform. I recognise her voice, with its American accent, from our phone call, but since she had mentioned she would be bringing her (breastfeeding) son with her, I hesitate – I had been waiting for a woman with a baby. I approach them as they are in the queue, discussing whether the child can have a chocolate doughnut (his preference) or a bran muffin (hers). I introduce myself, relieved to have found the right person, and we take a seat upstairs.

In the course of the next hour, Caroline bombards me with statistics. 'Did you know that 67 per cent of women in France have epidurals with their first baby? And 47 per cent with their second? Or that there is an 80 per cent episiotomy rate, and 30 per cent C-section rate? They are very into medicalised birthing here. They laugh at you if you say you want a natural birth. You're lucky in England.'

Once I explain my proposal, the conversation moves towards feeding. Caroline agrees that it's an important topic: France has one of the lowest breastfeeding rates in the world, she tells me. 'Seventy-five per cent of women say they wanted to breastfeed, but by the third day only 52 per cent are doing it. That's why La Leche's role is so crucial here. The health professionals know nothing about it, and the government doesn't care because they make so much money out of the formula manufacturers.' 'What was the group you mentioned?' I ask: 'La Leche League, like the one in the UK?'

'Yes, that's the breastfeeding support group I work with',[1] she says. 'No wonder the world is in such a state, with women so out of touch with their bodies. They're given the line about "breast is best", but given bottles in the hospital as soon as it gets tough. The bottle is so normalised that it's the global symbol for motherhood, even on toilet doors. So women don't get the support they really need. And then they get all resentful about people who promote breastfeeding, because of this chip on their shoulders saying that we are militant lactivists or whatever. I don't care if I'm militant! I almost didn't get help until it was too late with Louis. People need to know this stuff from the word go!'

Before I manage to ask more, she continues: 'It's the same with how long women go on feeding. We think that children should be weaned when it suits the mother. But it's only at 6 years old – 6 – that a child's need for breastmilk is finished. Only then that their immune system becomes independent. Which is why I still feed Louis.'

As if on cue, Louis lifts up her top and pulls at her bra. The man sipping his latte next to us looks surprised, to say the least. 'All right, darling', she says, 'don't hurt me, it's coming.' I do my best impression of nonchalance.

Looking back at my field notes a year later, I am amused by my shock.

This book profiles research with women in London and Paris who are members of La Leche League (LLL), an international breastfeeding support organisation founded in 1956 in the United States to support 'mothering through breastfeeding'. The text focuses on the accounts of a small but significant population of mothers within LLL who practise 'attachment mothering'. Attachment parenting – now a global movement with roots in the UK and the US – endorses parent-child proximity and typically involves long-term, on-cue breastfeeding, baby 'wearing' (Figure 0.1), and co-sleeping.

The endorsement of 'full-term' breastfeeding (up to eight years in the examples here, though typically for around three to four years) provides a case study by which to explore the recent 'intensification' of mothering. This trend is identified by a range of scholars writing about mothering in both the UK and the US (Arendell 2000; Avashai 2007; Bell 2004; Douglas and Michaels 2004; Duncan et al. 2003; Hays 1996; Lee 2007a, 2007b; Lee and Bristow 2009; Maher and Saugeres 2007; Milkie et al. 2004; Pugh 2005; Riggs 2005; Shaw 2008; Tronto 2009; Warner 2006), as well as beyond (Faircloth, Hoffman and Layne, forthcoming).

According to these scholars, the social role of mothering has expanded in recent years to encompass a range of tasks beyond the

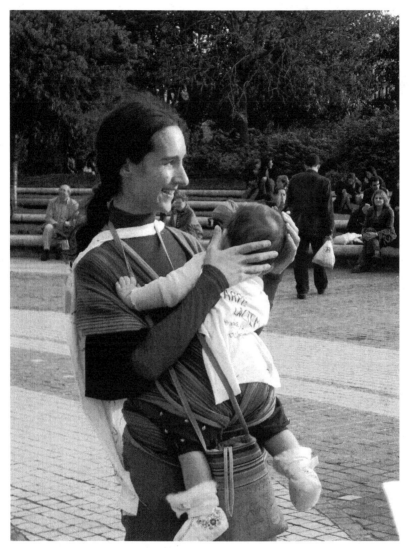

FIGURE 0.1. A mother wearing her baby in a sling at a 'nurse-in', Paris, October 2006, author's photo

straightforward rearing of children. Parents do much more than simply feed, clothe and shelter their children today, and it is this 'more' that is of interest here (Hays 1996: 5). The argument is that this new framework of 'intensive mothering' has meant that mothering is now understood to be a vehicle to personal fulfilment for women. This book therefore builds on and goes beyond traditional approaches to kinship in anthropology by looking at how related-ness is understood in conjunction with constructions of the self: for some women in this sample, being an (attachment) mother is akin to a vocation, and their primary nexus of what I refer to (after Goff-man 1959) as 'identity work'.

Breasts (and milk) are sites of multiple meaning, both as objects and as extensions of agency. Within anthropology and sociology, however, breastfeeding is generally explored either as a question of kinship (does it make us related?) or as a policy problem (why don't more women breastfeed?). The approach here is novel to the extent that breastfeeding is understood as an index of intensive mothering and a critical aspect of women's identity work. Of course feeding has long been central to the maternal identity, yet today, I argue, it is a particularly moralised affair. A strong orthodoxy (at the level of policy, at least) dictates that 'breast is best' – an injunction that affects women whether they breastfeed or not (Knaak 2005). To a very real extent, infant feeding is an embodied measure of moth-erhood (Sachs 2006), which has repercussions for virtually every other aspect of infant care (where the baby sleeps, who can care for it, etc.). In an era of 'informed choice', breastfeeding therefore operates as a highly moralised signifier dividing women into differ-ent camps along purported axes of child-centred or mother-centred forms of care.

Specifically, then, the book sets out to answer the questions of why and how infant feeding has become so tied to maternal iden-tity work. Certainly, individual choices are both visible and justified with reference to wider social patterns, but at the same time, infant feeding remains an acutely personal and accountable issue within mothering. Failure to breastfeed, amongst certain circles of women, can bring about a 'moral collapse' incomparable with 'failure' in other aspects of parenting (Lee 2008; see also Crossley 2009 for an auto-ethnographic perspective).

In taking their 'successful' (Avishai 2007, 2010) mothering prac-tices to an extreme with full-term breastfeeding, the women here invite critical engagement with their 'accountability strategies' (lit-erally, how they explain why they do what they do). Narratives are understood to be central to the construction of the self (see Miller 2005): in explaining their non-normative behaviour, these women provide commentary from the margins that prompts reflection on wider norms of maternal identity work and feeding. Whilst these women practice a form of infant feeding that is validated by wider policy directives emphasising the risks associated with formula milk use, their identity work is not as straightforward as may be expected. Indeed, women sit at a juncture between affirmation and opprobrium, highlighting a significant dissonance between statistical, ideological and cultural norms.

The accountability strategies women draw on (various forms of the natural, represented by evolution, science or instinct) already carry considerable cultural authority but are magnified by this group of mothers. The methodology used here, exploring both the stated rationales that women offer and observing the behaviour they display, dovetails into a discussion of 'accountability' (Strathern 2000). Throughout their narratives women both give their explicit rationalisations for full-term breastfeeding (their wish to ensure the health and well-being of their child) and reveal implicit intentions (tying this maternal duty to personal identity formation).

To explore the link between maternal identity work and infant feeding, I conducted long-term, in-depth fieldwork with women in LLL groups in London and Paris (both French-speaking and anglophone).[2] This fieldwork, conducted over the course of twelve months in 2006–07, provided the opportunity to follow women's experiences over an extended period of time, often from the early months of their child's life to well into the first year. This, in turn, allowed me to trace the evolution of particular women's attitudes towards infant feeding, which in some cases moved from moderate interest in establishing breastfeeding to passionate advocacy of full-term feeding. For the most part, the book focuses on the accounts of mothers; forthcoming research incorporates the accounts of fathers to 'triangulate' the parenting experience in the context of competing accountabilities in family life.

The term intensive mothering is used to refer to the general climate in which mothers (in the UK) currently raise their children (the argument later is that this climate is far less evident in France). Women in LLL may or may not internalise the injunction to mother intensively; where they do, they generally do so according to the 'attachment parenting' style, which is but one of many styles by which mothers care for their children intensively. Yet the attachment mothers focused upon here should not be taken as typical members of LLL – many women in the organisation do not show interest in the attachment parenting style of care or long-term breastfeeding. Those women I have classified as attachment mothers tend to be those who are most vocal, or 'militant' (as they sometimes put it) about the benefits of long-term breastfeeding, and it is their accounts that presented themselves most evidently for analysis.

A note on the title is therefore in order. Rather than being a statement about these mothers being 'militant lactivists', it is intended as a question seeking to understand why, how and with what implications such a label is used. As one attachment mother indicated, when it is used, 'it's fun because it's ironic. When others use it, it's not funny at all. It's insulting, because it ascribes a aggressive, combative, maliciousness to our behavior that doesn't exist.'

My own biography, of course, also plays a part in this account. One of the most frequent questions I am asked about the research is why I was interested in this subject at all, particularly as a woman without children. Much of my interest is shaped by my own mother, who happily describes herself – around the time that she gave birth to me, at least – as a 'clog-and-dungaree wearing hippy'. I was born at home, on a farm, and breastfed for nearly a year, which in 1982 was even more unusual than it might be now. My mother was a National Childbirth Trust educator, we used homeopathy to treat ailments in childhood, and many of my 'routine' vaccinations were delayed or avoided all together. Attachment parenting (and the associated values and practices) comes easily to me as I imagine how my own mothering might look.

Writing about the research has therefore inevitably been an exercise in writing about the self. Readers will no doubt recognise the tension inherent in anthropology, which sees researchers both participating in and objectifying social life. The process of reflection and analysis could sometimes be painful – I was forced to question things that had for so long seemed so straightforward (and that retain an 'affective' hold over me, even now). Issues faced by feminists, and feminism, became salient; Bobel's phrase 'bounded liberation' (2001) went some way towards describing the intersections of breastfeeding and 'empowerment' but also, as I discuss in the penultimate chapter, felt quite one-dimensional and problematic.

Doing Anthropology 'at Home'

Dangers attend anthropological research done in a familiar culture, as Richards's preface to Strathern's (1981) *Kinship at the Core* makes evident: cultural know-how can close down the potential for seeing the subtle differences which enlighten our accounts. In later work, Strathern complicates the bases of such concerns by differentiating the 'at-homeness' of anthropologist and informant. More than anything else, she says:

> What one must know is whether or not investigator/investigated are equally at home, as it were, with the kinds of premises about social life which inform anthropological enquiry. One suspects that whilst Travellers and Malay villagers [her examples of other sorts of anthropology done 'at home'] are not so at home, in their talk about 'community', 'socialization', or 'class', for example, Elmdoners are [referring to her work in an Essex village].... The personal credentials of the anthropologist do not tell us whether he/she is at home in this sense. But what he/she in the end writes, does: whether there is cultural continuity between the products of his/her labours and what people in the society being studied produce by way of accounts of themselves. (Strathern 1987: 17)

In doing anthropology at home, one does not simply hope to reproduce a script identical to those of one's informants. Indeed, the 'anthropological processing' (Strathern 1987: 17) that goes on means that our informants' accounts become 'data' that we overlay with analysis. There is therefore 'always a discontinuity between indigenous understandings and the analytical concepts which frame the ethnography itself' (Strathern 1987: 18). Mosse therefore calls ethnographic writing 'necessarily anti-social' (2006: 935) in that the inevitable split between field and desk (a distinction ever more muddy) leaves writing itself as the primary exit strategy from 'the field'.

So whilst anthropology at home involves a continuity between informants' cultural constructs and one's own, 'versions can always be challenged.... People may object to the value put on what they supply' (Strathern 1987: 26). This was certainly the case with my informants, who were unimpressed with an early conference presentation I made (which was posted on the organisers' website). The paper was an 'anthropological account' exploring the evolutionary claims around attachment parenting (an early version of Chapter 6 here). It differed from the anthropological accounts my informants had perhaps expected – that is, those that advocate parenting according to 'primitive' styles (e.g., biological anthropology or ethnographies of hunter-gatherer groups). My position as ethnographer was quite complex, then, in that I elicited accounts from my informants on the basis of expertise they assumed would validate their practices (despite no promises on this front); furthermore, my own sense of these assumptions as problematic was progressive.

Indicative of the global nature of the attachment parenting network, along with emails from LLL members and the chair of the LLL council in the UK, I received numerous emails from attachment parenting advocates in the United States (emphasis added):

Hello Ms. Faircloth,

... I live in the Los Angeles area, CA, USA. I am an active member
of LLL. I practice attachment parenting. I still breast feed my four-
and-a-half-year-old daughter, and we also co-sleep. I plan on doing
both those things until she is ready to stop. I was reading one of my
favorite websites, www.thecowgoddess.com when I came across a
link to your study. That website is run by a mother who is a fervent
supporter of anything attachment of [*sic*] natural parenting, and she
draws/writes comics on those topics. Her latest topic is your study,
which someone sent to her. Needless to say, the cow goddess, Hathor,
is greatly insulted by your study, as am I. It is very patronizing, to say
the least. *But, I do not have the energy to engage in an argument with you
over what I know in my heart, and is backed up by science, is doing the right
thing for my child.* I have however attached a link to an article from
the July 2003 issue of Mothering Magazine, which supports natural
family living [discussed in Chapter 7]. I often refer new moms, who
are looking for a way to validate their parenting philosophies on [*sic*]
their husbands or other family or friends, to this article. Read it and
take from it what you will.

sincerely,
[Name]

'Hathor'[3] is the creation of an artist, Heather Cushman-Dowdee, of
Los Angeles, California. As she writes on the site, the cow goddess is
'a superhero who wants to save humanity through the combination
of nurture, sustainability and bonding inherent in the practice of
attachment parenting. Her movement is called the Evolution Revolution, her breasts are her superpower and her sidekick is her baby,
always carried in a sling and prominently (politically) suckling at her
exposed breast ... Hathor is a mother who stays with her children
yet works as a woman of and ruling the world.' The website carried a
cartoon (Figure 0.2) of the 'Cow Goddess' reading out loud from my
presentation (which actually cites the work of Hausman 2003).

These emails – and many emails since – held a suggestion that
my work has disappointed LLL and the attachment parenting community by not advocating their practices more strongly (if at all).[4]
In fact, what irritated many commentators most was being unable
to work out whether it was 'for or against breastfeeding'. More than
one person suggested that as the author, I was 'anti-breastfeeding',
either because I did not have children or because I did and felt guilty
for not breastfeeding them. It could not be acknowledged that my
approach seeks to describe the conditions that make an intensive

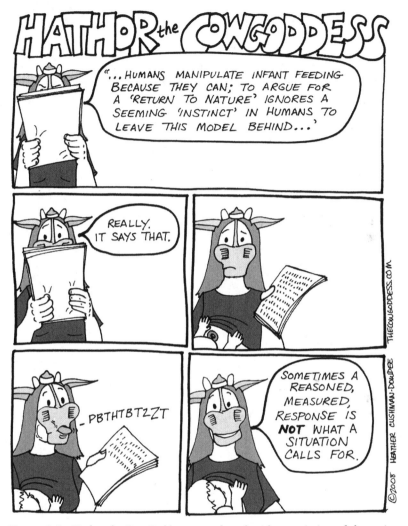

FIGURE 0.2. *Hathor the Cow Goddess*, reproduced with permission of the artist

commitment to one's child salient: there was no possibility but to be on one 'side' or the other. There was, to use Mosse's expression, a moral critique of my ethnographic exit (Mosse 2006: 946).

Doing the research therefore showed me that infant feeding is a peculiarly sensitive issue, given the way it relates to questions of maternal accountability and identity work. It is also one that has been deeply politicised. As one reader of an early draft of this text observed, a tension inheres in the personal practices of the women I worked with – who are individuals, doing what they want to do – and the role occupied by the organisations or networks to which they belong. In an advisory role to the government, LLL, for example, is actively engaged in shaping the maternity care women can expect to receive in the UK (and elsewhere). Whilst the women I worked with form an interesting anthropological study, the issue at the organisational level became more politically charged than I had ever anticipated. Due engagement with the particular knowledge claims presented in the name of breastfeeding advocacy therefore became increasingly pressing.

The cow goddess example helpfully reiterates that the accounts here are from women who are largely enthusiastic advocates of long-term breastfeeding. For many women, values and practices do not intersect in the same way as those of the women focused upon here: for countless mothers, long-term breastfeeding is just an intimate, pragmatic aspect of the mothering relationship, not a vehicle for public identity work mediated by politicised institutions such as LLL. For others, continuing to breastfeed is not a reflexive choice per se, but something they want to stop, yet feel unable to (for the sake of their child or otherwise). These jostling, entangled, emotional commitments are frequently screened out of the glossy narratives presented by advocates who are defensive about their long-term breastfeeding. Nevertheless, it is recognised that they are rarely far from the surface, and that they form the backdrop to women's accountability and identity work.

Summary

Chapter 1 of this volume provides a genealogy of intensive motherhood in the UK and explains the concept of identity work. The second chapter more closely explores the relationship between infant feeding and intensive motherhood, and intersections with government policy. Whilst many women claim to be 'marginal' with respect to their breastfeeding philosophies, this chapter shows that many attachment ideas are in fact quite mainstream and are increasingly being cemented in policy. Chapter 3 – to which readers largely interested in primary data analysis may wish to proceed directly – outlines the methodological approach taken and profiles the experiences of women who breastfeed to full term, highlighting the difficulty women can face in peer interactions when they continue to breastfeed their children for extended periods of time. For some women, LLL offers a haven from social criticism and isolation. The fourth and fifth chapters therefore outline the history and philosophy of LLL and attachment parenting more broadly, looking at how shared values create and sustain a sense of community.

Chapters 6, 7 and 8 look specifically at the accountability strategies women employ when rationalising their long-term breastfeeding (as evolutionarily natural, scientifically best and what feels right in their hearts). None of these strategies functions alone; rather, they work symbiotically to sustain women's identity work. Indeed, they serve as discursive threads that women weave together in the course of their narrativisation, operating both before and after the fact. In projecting these strategies into wider society, women edify group boundaries and validate their own choices in the creation of 'converts'. These chapters explore the slippage between description and prescription as a means of destabilising the authority of claims for the naturalness of full-term breastfeeding.

The final chapter – based on fieldwork in Paris – provides a contrast to illuminate the UK data. The argument is that in France as a whole, at the time of research, breastfeeding was not (yet) a public health issue, and there was not (yet) a culture of intensive parenting with a plethora of parenting 'options', nor (yet) a widespread validation of emotionally absorbing or 'natural' parenting practices, except amongst fringe groups that were accordingly more marginal. Mothering as an intensive activity and source of social identity was not validated to the same extent – indeed, *not* being too absorbed in one's child was considered desirable. This is denoted by a widely used vocabulary of '*esclavage*' (enslavement) to refer to breastfeeding, coupled with a caution against becoming a '*mère fusionelle*' (fused or over-attached mother). Such language is largely absent in the UK, at least in the early months of a baby's life.

This book's narrow focus on a nonconventional network of mothers provides opportunities for reflection on a wide range of anthropological topics, from kinship, identity and gender to accountability and knowledge claims. Women frequently cite anthropological studies of 'primitive' styles of breastfeeding as part of their rationalisations. Contextualising 'natural' grounds for behaviour has long been a disciplinary speciality, but in this case anthropology itself becomes anthropological object, forcing us to confront our own theoretical heritage.

Notes

1. Caroline was not speaking as a representative of LLL at this stage, though she was happy for me to use notes from our meeting in my research.
2. Fieldwork was approved by the Faculty Board of the Department of Social Anthropology in Cambridge, which subjected it to a full ethical review in line with the Association of Social Anthropologists' guidelines for ethical practice, retrieved from http://www.theasa.org/ethics.shtml Retrieved 22 November 2012 from ASA website. A Criminal Records Bureau check was also completed prior to the commencement of research.
3. Retrieved 14 March 2011 from http://www.thecowgoddess.com/rea soned-and-measured/ Page no longer exists, but available via: http://www.heathercushmandowdee.com/
4. Certainly not all mothers I met at LLL would align themselves with the label 'Evolution Revolution' – though there is a small population (within that population) who might. Meanwhile, it was interesting that in the twenty-nine comments left on the Cow Goddess website, several women mentioned their LLL groups (generally in the US). LLL itself would not condone Hathor, but neither would it object to her stance: her approach is too close to many of members' own.

Part I

THE CONTEXT OF CONTEMPORARY MOTHERING

Chapter 1

Intensive Motherhood and Identity Work

An Anthropology of Parenting?

Over the past twenty years in both the US and the UK, 'parenting' has emerged as a concept to describe the activity that parents do when raising children (Hoffman 2003, 2008). According to Furedi (2002), the transformation of the noun 'parent' into a verb, 'to parent', is a relatively recent phenomenon. First prominent in the 1950s in language used by psychologists, sociologists and self-help practitioners, it has subsequently spread into wider usage. Its popularity, in fact, can be seen in the extent to which 'parenting' has become a buzzword in policy circles: in 2007, the UK government unveiled its National Academy of Parenting Practitioners and published *Every Parent Matters* (Department for Education and Schools [DfES] 2007), a follow-up to the earlier *Every Child Matters* initiative (DfES 2003). More recently, the Minister of State for Children and Families announced a trial of 'universal parenting classes' for parents of children under five (Department for Education 2011).

At this wider political level, such discourses position the family as the source of – and solution to – a whole host of social ills, from poor educational outcome to recidivism. The sociologists Hays and Furedi argue that the emergence of parenting also needs to be seen as part of a larger social commentary about the family 'at risk' or 'in crisis'. The health and safety of children is increasingly seen as compromised by a toxic social environment (Furedi 2002). This inflated sense of risk, Furedi argues, opens the door to increased surveillance and policy advice. Indeed, parenting has acquired a particular place in contemporary societies, where the burden of managing risks in-creasingly devolves onto individuals and families (Hoffman 2008, see also Lee et al., forthcoming).

For parents themselves, then, parenting is not just a new word for child-rearing. Rather, it requires a specific skill set: a certain level of expertise about children and their care, based on the latest re-search on child development, as well as an affiliation to a certain way of raising a child, by any one of a number of available methods (whether Gina Ford, attachment or otherwise). Being well educated is a requirement for participation in these choices, as is a certain access to economic resources. As Hoffman says, however: "Most of all [parenting] means being both discursively positioned by and ac-tively contributing to the networks of ideas, values, practices and social relations that have come to define a particular form of the politics of parent-child relations within the domain of the contem-porary family" (Hoffman 2008).

Parenting is, of course, heavily gendered. Phoenix, Wollett and Lloyd note that the feminist movement of the 1970s included argu-ments that women should not shoulder the entire burden for in-fant care. Mothering became parenting in a bid to be more inclusive – although, as they put it, 'ideas about "parenthood" as something gender free began to emerge as "questionable"' (Phoenix, Wollett and Lloyd 1991: 4). 'Parenthood' obscures the reality that 'mothers are still the people who do most childrearing and have most responsi-bility for children, [and] any examination of parenting has to take seriously this gender differentiation and the ways in which it is un-derpinned by power relations' (Phoenix, Wollett and Lloyd 1991: 5). For this reason, I chose to refer to 'intensive motherhood' and 'mothering' here, whilst recognising that fathers are also influenced (albeit in different ways) by these shifts in wider parenting culture (Dermott 2008; Featherstone 2009).

Accordingly, in *The Cultural Contradictions of Motherhood*, Hays (1996) explores how mothers are encouraged to parent their chil-dren intensively. Based on her research with working mothers in the United States, she argues that intensive motherhood is an emer-gent ideology that urges mothers to 'spend a tremendous amount of time, energy and money in raising their children' (Hays 1996: x). Hays suggests that this injunction remains culturally salient, de-spite an uneasy relationship with the logic of the workplace, both because it props up the capitalist infrastructure and because mother-ing is perceived as 'the last best defence against what many people see as the impoverishment of social ties, communal obligations and unremunerated commitments' (Hays 1996: xiii). This, in turn, has had a profound impact on the way adults experience parenthood (Douglas and Michaels 2004; Furedi 2002).

Yet the ways in which parents' experiences have been affected by an era of intensive parenting – in short, the transformation of 'parent' from a noun to a verb – is not a topic, so far, that has been explored significantly within the anthropological discipline. Hoffman notes that in the emergence of parenting as a distinctive approach to child-rearing, the negotiation of authority, power and social control is mediated by networks of professional expertise and shared knowledge/practice. Parenting as 'public culture' is thus problematic for the anthropologist because it is constituted by individuals (experts, parents), networks (mother-communities, parenting groups), institutions (academies, organisations), media (Internet, film, TV, books, magazines) and other forms of knowledge production (research, journalism, popular and academic information and analysis). Furthermore, parenting is both lived experience and an object of academic enquiry: to some extent, we have all experienced parenting. This curious public/private relationship however means that an anthropological perspective has a particularly significant role to play.

This book investigates the experiential dimension of this historical shift. In particular, it explores the identity work of a sample of nonconventional mothers, who intensify further the injunction to parent intensively by investing large amounts of time and energy in raising their children. As noted, there are many ways of caring for children intensively (e.g., methods that advocate the strict timetabling of feeding, sleeping etc., which indeed are just as prevalent as the attachment parenting focused on here). The philosophy of attachment parenting, which validates attentive, embodied care for infants, offers women *one* set of norms by which to structure their identity work in congruence with an overarching framework of intensive mothering. This framework holds both points of congruence and points of departure, as I will show.

This chapter opens by positioning parenting within anthropological work on kinship before outlining some characteristics of an intensive mothering framework. In short, optimal childcare is presented as being child-centred and expert-guided. The discussion historicises each of these facets before closing with an exploration of a particularly notable aspect of intensive mothering: mothering as a space for women's identity work, a nexus through which they position themselves as social agents.

Parenting and / as Kinship

This project is not a traditional study of kinship in the sense of trying to understand *how* people consider themselves related – that
is, through nature, culture or otherwise. (In fact, consideration of
breastfeeding would complicate the very basis of these discussions, in
that it is a practice by which people consider themselves, in the UK at
least, to be *physiologically* – that is, neither simply genetically nor simply socially – related. This is not a form of relatedness that translates
easily into idioms of British kinship, or into our legal framework.)

Yet the book certainly draws on a tradition within kinship studies that aims to problematise the stability of those very categories
(Strathern 1993). Drawing on examples from the Artificial Reproductive Technologies, Strathern argues that nature can no longer be
considered the grounding for culture, simply there to be 'discovered'
– it is, she says, partly produced through technological innovation of
what had previously remained implicit. At the same time, these categories remain powerful in the public imagination (and it is interesting that the women in this sample do look to one version of nature
as a grounding for culture, as I discuss later). Kinship remains particularly important for Euro-Americans, she says, because it is a domain where nature and culture are held to interconnect (see also
Franklin and McKinnon 2001; Ragoné 1994; Rapp 2000).

Furthermore, that kinship confers obligations and is about the
creation of social personhood, is certainly central here. As Loizos
and Heady (1999) say, 'Kinship can be thought of in terms of moral
obligations and rights. Some of the most important proceed down-
ward from parent to child and, subsequently, upward from child to
parent. Who must feed whom?' (Loizos and Heady 1999: 5). Perhaps more pragmatically, then, the subject of interest here is what
Goody refers to as the 'affective' obligations of kinship, as much as
the jural ones it also confers: 'While jural rights in, and duties with
respect to, children are clearly important, the affective ties between
parents and their children, parents' role in socialisation and education, and the claims which can be made in the name of morality are
also highly significant, and they are certainly subject to a wide range
of transactions' (Goody 1982: 7).

So to argue for an anthropology of parenting is not to suggest a
move away from kinship per se. Indeed, it is 'relatedness' (Carsten
2000) that makes parenting a morally loaded occupation for adults.
In *Kinship, Law and the Unexpected*, Strathern (2005) uses a vignette
drawn from the work of Miller, who worked with mothers in National Childbirth Trust (NCT) groups in North London. He illustrates

how mothers are occupied by risk avoidance and optimisation after the birth of their children, the means of which are a subject of constant debate. Strathern observes:

> the young mother is placed in a position of responsibility *by her knowledge of* the effects of these substances and toys on the growing body, and on the growing mind and sets of behaviours ... the child seems to embody the conscientiousness with which the mother has acted on her knowledge and stuck to her principles ... its development reflects the application of her own knowledge. (Strathern 2005 4–5, emphasis in original)

Why is this so critical for the mother? Strathern notes that a parent shares a body with the child twice over:

> First is the body of genetic inheritance, a given, a matter regarded colloquially as of common blood or common substance. Second is the body that is a sign of the parent's devotion – or neglect – and it is in this middle class milieu above all through the application of knowledge that the parent's efforts make this body ... [Miller] jokes that the child grows the mother. (Strathern 2005: 5)

Taking this focus on the affective relationship between mother and child, this study therefore looks specifically at processes of maternal self-formation – that is, how relatedness is understood in women's constructions of themselves.

In emails, for example, many of my informants' addresses represented their family status (*Charlotte@Brookfamily.net*), or bore more specific names such as *Lactivist@ecoparents.co.uk*.[1] In email signatures, some mothers embellished their status by specifying what type of mother they were – 'Attachment parent to Elsie, 2'; 'On-demand breastfeeder to Rose, 19 months'; 'Co-sleeper to Emily and Zachary, 5 and 3' and so forth – often providing a link to a website supporting such practices below the name. This is one example of what I refer to as 'mothering as identity work'. For Radcliffe-Brown (1952), kin terms paralleled the distribution of the ego's rights and duties. The terms here are not so much about cultivating rights and duties in the ego; they are appropriated and magnified by mothers *as* mothers in the course of their identity work.

The UK Context

In the UK, private and public health care systems work in parallel. The National Health Service provides free (or nearly free) treatment for all citizens, including all perinatal care. Private health care is also available, though at considerably greater cost, typically involving clients' paying for an insurance policy to cover the cost of care.

Women usually have their pregnancies confirmed by their GP (general practitioner), who registers them with a midwife. The first meeting with the midwife takes place either in a hospital, or at a community practice (a health centre, GP surgery or at home). The midwife performs a series of tests and checks, and advises women on local antenatal classes to help prepare for birth and life with a baby. A range of checks is performed throughout women's pregnancies, with the first 'dating' scan typically between ten and fourteen weeks. A considerable amount of information about infant feeding and care is passed on at this point, and throughout the rest of the pregnancy.

The majority of babies in the UK are born in hospital or 'midwife-led units', though so-called low-risk women are also offered the option of home birth (around 2 percent of births are currently at home, Birth Choice UK, 2011). Women are encouraged to bring along a 'birth plan' outlining their preferences for treatment during their time in hospital (NHS 2009). Midwives handle most routine births, whilst obstetricians are on call in hospitals to help with complications. Women usually only stay one or two nights in hospital (unless they have had a caesarean section delivery) and in that time are offered support and information about infant feeding and general care. Following a mother's discharge from hospital, a 'health visitor' sees her at home in the first few days after birth. During these visits, both mother and baby are checked for any abnormalities, and the baby is weighed to ensure normal patterns of growth. At a six-week postnatal check, women may also be screened for postnatal depression. Mothers may make continued visits to a 'baby clinic' to monitor their child's growth. Breastfeeding exclusively for six months is encouraged, and many outlets offer women support to this end, including LLL, the Association of Breastfeeding Mothers, the National Childbirth Trust and the Breastfeeding Network.

Intensive Mothering

Methods of childcare can be divided into those styles that are 'structured', and those that are (putatively, at least) 'unstructured'. The former might be characterised by scheduled feeding, formula feeding and separate sleeping. Unstructured models, by contrast, aim to dissolve notions of rational efficiency in favour of more relaxed styles of care, often characterised by practices like long-term, on-cue breastfeeding, a family bed and 'positive' discipline (Buskens 2001: 75).[2]

Of course, the distinction between the models may be more heuristic than descriptive, as many parents will attest, since one can adopt characteristic elements of one style (e.g., breastfeeding) and deploy them as part of the other (e.g., on schedule, as part of separate sleeping). Similarly, there may be a gap between intention and outcome (formula feeding being not always a deliberate, reflexive choice but sometimes a necessary intervention when breastfeeding is problematic). But because the plurality exists, at a heuristic level at least, parents are accountable for the choices they make both within and between these models. In Foucault's language, in contemporary liberalism the responsible moral actor is not one who conforms blindly to expert or even popular recommendations. 'Rather, she is expected to subject such recommendations to evaluation and questioning, operating as an informed consumer' (Murphy 2003: 457). Following Strathern, this is a heavily moralised affair: those who are not reflexive, informed consumers are deemed irresponsible or in need of education.

The argument here is that whichever way an 'informed' woman in the UK chooses to mother, she must now do so intensively. Lee and Bristow (2009) identify two major characteristics of intensive mothering: (1) mothering is defined as a practice that should be child-centred, and (2) mothers should pay attention to what experts say about their children. They both have instrumental effects with respect to knowledge and practice.

Child-Centred Care

To say a child's interests should be placed before the mother's is, perhaps, not anything remarkable – indeed, Douglas has said that the 'absolute morality' of motherhood is that 'in all circumstances, babies take precedence over mothers' (Douglas, in Murphy 1999: 200). But the way in which this injunction is realised is certainly novel. Hays notes that today, children are not to be excluded from adult leisure time but 'listened to' and 'included'. Weekend activities, for example, should centre around maximising children's health and well-being, and mothers are expected to act as pseudo-teachers, optimising their children's intelligence through a range of extracurricular activities (Hays 1996). The attachment mothers I focus on here certainly internalise this aspect of the intensive motherhood ideology – like many other mothers – by placing their children at the centre of their parenting strategies.

Indeed, the mother's role has expanded dramatically in recent years, not least because psychologists' interest in early infancy burgeoned in the 1950s. The idea that experience during infancy determines the course of future development, and therefore that parental intervention determines the future fate of a youngster, has had a profound effect on the way parents structure their relationships with their offspring. Furedi argues about these 'myths' that 'by grossly underestimating the resilience of children, they intensify parental anxiety and encourage excessive interference in children's lives; by grossly exaggerating the degree of parental intervention required to ensure normal development, they make the task of parenting impossibly burdensome' (Furedi 2002: 45). This focus on parents reduces the agency of children themselves, meanwhile eclipsing the effect of peers and social climate on child development. Accordingly, a highly interventionist approach is legitimised on the parents' part, and the importance of the parenting role increases in congruence.

With studies stressing the importance of the early (even pre-conception) environment for infant development (see Gerhardt 2004), providing children with the right kind of environment turns normal parenting activities into a series of tasks to be achieved. Touching, talking and feeding are no longer ends in themselves, but tools mothers are required to perfect to ensure optimal development. Lee, Macvarish and Bristow (2010) give the example of playing with a child: no longer simply an enjoyable activity for adult and child, it has become an instrumental way of ensuring positive long-term outcomes. The everyday experience of mothering is re-written as set of skills to be honed and perfected if one is to achieve optimum development (Rose 1999).

Rose has even argued that love can be used to promote a certain type of self-understanding in children, and is duly emphasised for mothers as increasing confidence, helpfulness and dependability at the same time that it averts fear, cruelty or any other deviation from the desired norm (Rose 1999: 160). The conversion of love from a spontaneous sentiment manifested in warm affection into a parental function or skill is one of the key reasons mothers are now routinely told 'Enjoy your baby' with almost magical powers ascribed to unconditional love (Furedi 2002: 79).

The understood irreversibility of a kinship tie with a child leaves parents little room for manoeuvre here – because all decisions about a child's care rest squarely on parental shoulders, any mistake is perceived as liable to ruin the child's chances in life. This rather gloomy picture is but a logical outcome, 'when one interlocks loving a child with feeling responsible for its welfare and being uncertain how to achieve this – a plight rich in poignancy and disasters all of its own' (Beck and Beck-Gernsheim 1995: 119).

Expertise

The second aspect of intensive mothering – that mothers should re- fer to experts when caring for their child – is also intimately tied up with the expansion of the parental role. In *Paranoid Parenting* (2002), Furedi argues that parenting is increasingly considered too important a job to be left to parents themselves to deal with. Lee (2007b) suggests that this, in turn, binds mothering to the job of risk management, at once creating and fuelling the market for a plethora of experts who 'enable' mothers to avoid certain risks and optimise their children (whether these experts be judo teachers, osteopaths or psychologists, to use just some of Hays's examples). This outsourc- ing of authority has the potential to reduce parental confidence, says Furedi, to the extent that all parents are tinged with some degree of paranoia (Furedi 2002; see also Ramaekers and Suissa 2011). As I explore later, the mothers I work with consider themselves the ex- perts on their own children and talk about following their instincts as a means of countering this anxiety (although it is interesting that these 'instincts' are often clarified after contact with 'experts' in LLL or encountered in their wider reading).

Writing about the US, Apple notes that the development of ex- pert knowledge about mothering was intimately tied up with the ra- tional-efficient management of birth and infant care, which became increasingly prevalent during the twentieth century (Apple 1987). With the increasing hospitalisation of birth, measurements concern- ing infant development were collected by medical staff and observed over time, with norms duly calculated. These measurements were taken under the auspices of enabling women to optimise their child's development. The scales that physicians used in the medicalisation of maternity were not just 'measures,' however. They provided *new* ways to think about mothering and created a logical gap between the expectation and the observed (Rose 1999).

Scholars who have analysed the 'accountability culture' within both finance and other areas of social life (Hoskin 1996; Power 1994; Strathern 1997, 2000) comment that since measures only report 'what is', they are seemingly unobjectionable. But in fact, they also prescribe what 'ought' to be in the form of conscious or unconscious targets, in the guise of only being 'for the best' (Hoskin 1996: 267). Where there is deviation from the norm, measures are justified on the basis of preserving, or improving, that very norm. Marking an important shift in the politics of family life, experts (social workers, practitioners etc.) were afforded the right to intervene if the child was seen to be endangered, or even potentially endangered. The images of normality generated by expertise also have a final function, as a means by which individuals can themselves normalise and evaluate their lives.

Intensive Motherhood: A 'Local Moral World'

In his preface to *A Contribution to the Critique of Political Economy*, Marx describes ideology: 'The totality of … relations of production constitutes the economic structure of society, the real foundation, on which arises a legal and political superstructure and to which correspond definite forms of social consciousness … it is not the consciousness of men that determines their existence, but their social existence that determines their consciousness' (Marx 1977: 20).

Ideology, he argues, is generated by – and does the job of – justifying an exploitative economic base (in a capitalist mode of production). As part of what he refers to as the superstructure, ideology is at once deceptive, in that it masks the real nature of economic relations, and reflective, in that it is generated by that exploitative base. Ideology sustains individuals living within particular economic realities by giving them a masked view of the world, thereby quelling potential discontent. As Bloch (1989) argues succinctly, ideologies both reflect *and* hide the world.

Hays refers to intensive motherhood as an emergent ideology, as it goes some way towards 'propping up' the public/private split inherent to the capitalist mode of production. Yet women who enter the labour market, she points out, are in a historically novel contradiction in that they are torn between two competing ways of being: rational efficiency at work, and intensive mothering at home.[3] Far from diluting the contradiction, as one might expect, women's entry into the market has taken place in parallel with an increasing emphasis the importance of labour-intensive, emotionally absorbing mothering. The language of 'juggling' is – in the UK at least – now commonplace.

The attachment mothers discussed here tend to cease (or certainly reduce) employed labour in the early years of their child's life. Whilst these women do not therefore on a daily basis embody the 'cultural contradiction' that Hays describes, they nevertheless remain subject to the more pervasive social values intensive mothering engenders and sustains: that is, that mothering is in logical opposition to the marketplace, and that children are quite literally 'priceless' (Zelizer 1985). As Schneider observes about the US:

> The contrast between home and work brings out aspects which complete the picture of the distinctive features of kinship in American culture…. Indeed, what one does at home, it is said, one does for love, not for money, while what one does at work one does strictly for money, not for love. Money is material, it is power, it is impersonal and universalistic, unqualified by considerations of sentiment and morality…. Love on the other hand is highly personal, and particularistic, and beset with considerations of sentiment and morality. (Schneider 1969: 119)

I deliberately refer to intensive motherhood not as a 'hegemonic idea' of appropriate mothering but as an 'emergent ideology'. I take the distinction from the Comaroffs' *Of Revelation and Revolution* (1991), where the former is understood to 'refer to that order of signs and practices, relations and distinctions, images and epistemologies – drawn from a historically situated cultural field – that comes to be taken for granted as the natural and received shape of the world', and the latter is 'an *articulated* system of meanings, values and beliefs of a kind that can be abstracted as [the] worldview of any social grouping' (Comaroff and Comaroff 1991: 23–24, emphasis added). As they put it: 'The first is nonnegotiable and therefore beyond direct argument; the second is more susceptible to being perceived as a matter of inimical opinion and interest and therefore is open to contestation. Hegemony homogenizes, ideology articulates' (Comaroff and Comaroff 1991: 24). Intensive mothering is an ideology of appropriate mothering in that it forms the subject of public debate about 'family values' and maternity policies. To say that women are subject to an ideology of intensive mothering is not to suggest they are 'duped' or 'falsely conscious' – indeed, the women I worked with are highly reflexive. Instead, this term is used to expose how these ideas have such cultural purchase at the same time that they are articulated as problematic.

The status of motherhood has inflated, then – not diminished – as women have continued to enter the labour market. Yet Phoenix, Wollett and Lloyd note that the relationship between motherhood and employed work is a critical one, not only because it props up the capitalist infrastructure, but also because it provides women with an opportunity for identity work reminiscent of a career, that is, an alternative to the labour market:

> In addition to establishing women's credentials as women, [motherhood] also provides women with an occupational and structural identity because it takes up a great deal of women's time and energy and can be a substitute for involvement in other activities, such as employment. ... How motherhood is understood and hence how women view themselves as mothers is very much part of the historical period and ideological circumstances in which ideas develop. (Phoenix, Wollett and Lloyd 1991: 6)

In summarising the characteristics of intensive motherhood, Hays argues that 'the methods of appropriate child-rearing are constructed as *child-centred, expert-guided, emotionally absorbing, labour intensive, and financially expensive*' (Hays 1996: 8, emphasis in original). Drawing on Kleinman (1995), we might say that intensive motherhood constitutes a 'local moral world' in that it enables mothers to narrate their practices in culturally specific, meaningful ways:

> [M]oral accounts are the commitments of social participants in a local world about what is at stake in everyday experience ... the contexts and processes of moral life involve more than individuals. They also are based in collective orientations, social resources, and intersubjective action. The moral is actualized not only in subjective space but in social transactions over what locally matters, often virtually so, such as marriages, family, work, child rearing, education, religious practice, health and death. Conflicts among different priorities create moral dilemmas as social problems that require action. (Kleinman 1995: 45)

Intensive motherhood presents a paradigm of *ideal* motherhood, then. This is not to say that all women endorse (or practise) all aspects of this paradigm. Rather than being a uniform set of practices, intensive motherhood is 'the normative standard ... by which mothering practices and arrangements are evaluated' (Arendell 2000: 1195).

To be reflexive about knowledge is a largely middle-class concern in the UK (Strathern 2005: 3), and the focus on intensive motherhood is to take a specifically middle-class angle here. Although this is discussed at length in Chapter 3, where the demographic profile of interviewees is presented, Hays's argument is followed to the extent that engagement with this framework of intensive mothering is valuable because it presents culturally dominant beliefs. That is, the middle class presents the most powerful, visible and self-consciously articulated model readily apparent in public discourse and policy. Strathern says in *After Nature,* her examination of English kinship, that 'I focus on middle-class usage [of kinship terms], largely to do with the way the middle class enunciate and communicate what they regard as general social values' (Strathern 1992b: 25).

Historicising Intensive Motherhood

Across space and time, societies have had different ideas about children, which in turn shape how parents are expected to behave towards them. As Mead observed, 'Primitive materials ... give no support to the theory that there is a "natural" connection between conditions of human gestation and delivery and appropriate cultural beliefs' (1962: 54). And drawing on the work of authors such as Ariès (1962), Badinter (1981), and Hardyment (1995), it is clear that the view of children we take today is highly specific.

Badinter and Ariès, writing about Europe in the Middle Ages, describe how children were understood to be 'gluttonous beasts' by their parents, useless until they could be put to work at around the age of seven (although see Wilson [1980] for a critique of this). During the sixteenth and seventeenth centuries – and indicative of what might be termed a broader 'parent-centred' approach – women who could afford to do so typically sent their children to wet nurses in the provinces (Fildes 1986). Certainly, any suggestion that mothering (or fathering) were activities in which adults would find emotional and personal fulfilment was absent, at least in public discourse.

Around the eighteenth century this picture in Europe began to change, these authors argue, as represented in the writings of Rousseau and the publication of his *Emile* (1762). The idea of childhood as a valuable period of life, and the child as something sacred and noble, was expounded in wider Enlightenment thinking. Prioritising the child's needs, Rousseau argued that maternal practices should 'follow from the development of a child's inner nature, rather than from adult interests, and that children should be cherished, treated with love and affection, and protected from the corruption of the larger society' (Rousseau in Hays 1996: 26). In particular, he advised women to 'look to the animals' for their examples of appropriate infant care, arguing that women should breastfeed their own children, a campaign that was enthusiastically taken up by an influential group of French noblewomen (Blaffer Hrdy 2000).

Hays argues that rather than a pendulum swing between different styles of childcare (crudely, from parent-centred to child-centred and back again until the present day), a gradual *intensification* of motherhood occurred during the nineteenth century. It was during this time, she argues, that some of the most enduring features of the intensive motherhood framework were crystallised. Mothers, for instance, became valorised as keepers of morality, transmuted via the care they were encouraged to lavish on their children. Where once large families were preferable, during the nineteenth and twentieth centuries family size decreased dramatically, with each child becoming more precious in the process. Phoenix, Wollett and Lloyd (1991) pinpoint this as the era in Europe in which motherhood became cemented as a social role, again with ramifications for the present day: 'The word "motherhood" emerged as a concept in Victorian times when it was reified as being motherliness, of mothering. ... Motherhood is now usually considered to be an essential task or stage of women's development as well as a crucial part of their identity, often from childhood' (Phoenix, Wollett and Lloyd 1991: 6).

Hardyment saw the era as characterised by a curious mix of 'science and sentimentality' (1995: 147). Similarly, writing about the US, Apple (2006) has argued that 'scientific parenting', the trend she most associates with twentieth-century parenting, eclipsed maternal authority in conjunction with the promotion of 'modern' parenting methods (what I term 'structured' care, although 'unstructured' models today also rely on scientific validation). This modern, rational-efficiency message was echoed, she argues, in books, pamphlets, by public health nurses, and in educational trailers, all with a view to building healthy citizens. In the early 1900s, Truby-King was the most influential advocate of this 'scientific' style of care in the UK, promoting practices such as scheduled sleeping and formula feeding, with the aim of creating physically and morally well-adjusted citizens of the empire. Apple argues that whilst these methods were introduced with the aim of improving infant health and reducing mortality, they had the additional effect of alienating the mother from her baby. The widespread hospitalisation of birth during the late twentieth century meant that these practices of separation became normalised and widespread, and introduced a relationship between motherhood and expert knowledge that remains evident to this day (that is, whilst a mother is entirely responsible for her child, she should consult experts on how to go about enacting this duty).

For a small elite, some of the scientific model promoted by the likes of Truby-King fell out of favour during the 1930s, and strict rules about handling and feeding babies started to lose popularity. The Aldriches published *Babies Are Human Beings* in 1938 (Hardyment 1995: 213), encouraging women to let their children determine feeding and eating patterns in a more 'unstructured' approach (following the outbreak of war in the UK, this was more widely taken up in the US). Hays argues that childcare became child-centred in this period, noting that 'the most striking feature of [this] advice is the idea that the natural development of the child and the fulfilment of children's desires are needs in themselves and should be the fundamental basis of child-rearing practices' (Hays 1996: 45).

Establishing that mothers should follow the lead of their children did not quell the search for expertise, however – indeed, children, it was argued, must have their needs interpreted by experts, who could guide parents in turn. More and more manuals on child-rearing began to appear. It was also during this period that the categories of psychological and cognitive child development came into vogue: Freud (1977), Erikson (1959) and Piaget (1955) published studies of childhood, associating childhood experience with adult development.

What linked these studies was the understanding of the absolute necessity of a mother's loving nurture. Animal studies became the basis for arguments about the importance of maternal attachment. Some of the first work in this area was done by Lorenz (1937, 1950), who introduced the term imprinting to refer to a phenomenon of an 'attachment window.' The basic principle was demonstrated by studies on ducklings conducted by Hess (1966), whereby ducklings were shown to form an attachment to whichever caretaker they first came into contact with (Gardner 1997). The argument was that a child's first hours, weeks and months of life had a lasting impact on the entire course of the child's development (see for example Klaus and Kennell 1976). By the 1980s it was argued that a child's development would be put at risk if the mother had failed to 'bond' immediately after birth (Furedi 2002: 53). Despite there being, in fact, little clinical evidence in support of this theory (Eyer 1992, also see chapter 7), this idea has remained hugely influential.

Attachment theory claimed that the constant presence of a loving and responsive attachment figure – typically the mother – was the foundation for lifelong mental health. On the basis of his research with children in institutional settings, the psychiatrist and psychoanalyst Bowlby wrote in 1952: 'What is believed to be essential for mental health is that the infant and young child should experience a warm, intimate and continuous relationship with his mother (or permanent mother-substitute) in which both find satisfaction and enjoyment.... A state of affairs in which the child does not have this relationship is termed "maternal deprivation"' (Bowlby 1995: 11). It was into this context that the wealth of experts we know today (Spock, Leach and Brazelton, to name three of the most popular spanning the last half of the twentieth century) produced the first editions of books designed to help parents parent.

The language of enablement sat well within the discourse of 'enjoying' parenting and 'trusting yourself' (the famous first words of Spock's *Baby and Child Care,* published in 1946). Implicitly, the authors of these texts share the view that childcare is the responsibility of the mother, that methods should be child-centred (but guided by experts), and that children (and their care) are outside of marketplace valuation (Hays 1996: 52). As Hays notes, Leach's book is written almost entirely from the child's point of view. The implication by these three authors is that mothers are irreplaceable in the caregiving relationship (that is, third parties such as fathers or nannies cannot be trusted to do a good enough job). Interviewed in 1988, Brazelton discusses whether mothers should stay at home to look after their children. 'Does the first year really make a difference?' asks the interviewer. 'It does', Brazelton says. 'The child gets a sense of being important ... if he doesn't have that through infancy, it's hard to put it in later ... and these kids will become difficult in school ... they'll become delinquents later and eventually they'll become terrorists.'[4] Anyone that does undertake the task in lieu of the mother should be verified and monitored by the mother.

Today, experts appear to have reworked 'scientific' motherhood for the contemporary age with a range of neuroscientifically inspired books. Interestingly, these books, such as Gerhardt's *Why Love Matters: How Affection Shapes a Baby's Brain,* appear to reject 'modern' parenting and return to more 'traditional' (supposedly primitive and instinctual) styles of care, again with a stress on the importance of maternal care (see Chapter 6).

Reading advice manuals is, of course, not a direct reflection of actual practices amongst women in their own homes. However, such advice enables academics to gauge what was considered beneficial for raising healthy children. Similarly, not all women are affected by advice in the same way – they negotiate it according to other constraints in their lives (Beck and Beck-Gernsheim 1995). Yet it is notable that Spock's *Baby and Child Care* remains a worldwide best-seller (outsold only by the Bible) – indicating clearly considerable congruence with what women are actually doing, or at least what they think they should be doing. Hardyment (1995) concludes *Perfect Parents: Baby-Care Advice Past and Present* with a section entitled 'Spotlight on Parents' that highlights how parenting has become particularly visible in the public eye, and is ever more tied up with adults' quest for a 'sense of self', or what I term identity work.[5] She shows how widespread knowledge of these patterns of behaviour not only enabled mothers to assess the development of their children but also introduced an element of competition, leaving women 'feeling more inadequate than ever' (Hardyment 1995: 197).

Mothering as Identity Work: Narrative Processes of Self-Making

Anthropologically, the theoretical interest in this text is novel in proposing an engagement with mothering as identity work. This is partly a product of historical circumstance: only recently has mothering been an identity that women can work at (Arendell 2000; Avishai 2007, 2010; Lee and Bristow 2009).

The concept of identity has a long trajectory in the social sciences (see, e.g., Giddens 1991; Jenkins 1996; Mead 1934; Strathern 1992b; Stryker 1968), where the term is typically used to denote an individual's comprehension of selfhood. In particular, these accounts have focused on the ways in which individuals (and indeed groups) constitute their identity in negotiation with wider society. For Stryker (1968), for example, the purpose of 'identity negotiation' (between the individual and society) is to develop a consistent set of behaviours that reinforce the identity of the person within the wider social context.

Many of the discussions around identity have aimed at de-stabilising the notion that it is a natural, fixed or objective criteria, asserting that identity itself is instead a political project in which individuals and groups engage in accordance with social and historical contingencies (Giddens 1991). In their critique of identity as a concept, Brubaker and Cooper (2000) note that there remains a tendency in scholarly writing to confuse identity as a category of practice and as a category of analysis, leaving it a somewhat ill-defined term floating between the poles of reification and ambiguity.

For this reason the focus here is on identity work rather than on identity per se. This is intended to highlight the active processes by which identity is constructed, as well as the inherently social nature of this enterprise (as opposed to it being simply a means of self-expression). Thus, whilst identity itself may be an abstract entity, its manifestations and the ways it is exercised are often open to view: in language, dress, behaviour, use of space and so forth. During social encounters individuals assert elements of their identity through these mechanisms; in this sense identity work refers to the range of *activities* in which individuals engage to create, present and sustain personal identities, with particular reference to the constitution of relatedness (Goffman 1959).

Specifically, women's identity work is examined in the accounts they articulated during interviews or in questionnaires concerning their infant feeding practices (and specifically, long-term breastfeeding). Many scholars have emphasised the role of language in the constitution of personhood, arguing 'that human beings actually live out their lives as 'narratives', [and] that we make use of the stories of the self that our culture makes available to us to plan out our lives ... to account for events and give them significance, to accord ourselves an identity' (Rose 1999: xviii). For Beck and Beck-Gernsheim (1995), our biographies are increasingly choice biographies. In the contemporary age, they argue, we must reflexively make our own narratives as traditional structures such as class, gender and racial constraints fall away.

'Accounting' – literally, the act of giving accounts – means simply explaining why you are doing what you are doing. Far from being removed from everyday sociality, as notions of financial accounting might imply, accountability is always going on: 'Whether in what we say, or by what we do, we are always giving explanations and reasons for our conduct' (Munro and Mouritsen 1996: 4). Accountability – in the sense of rendering intelligible some aspect of our selves – 'is a distinctive and pervasive feature of what it is to be human' (Munro and Mouritsen 1996: 23). It is a condition of our participation in our social world. And it is a particularly prominent aspect of women's experiences of infant feeding, a heavily surveilled domain in both formal and informal terms. It is in this respect that women's accountability strategies are referred to here, as they rationalise their unusual practices in the highly moralised arena of infant feeding. This accounting, in turn, effects a certain sort of self. Drawing on Adam Smith:

> When I endeavour to examine my own conduct ... it is evident that, in all such cases, I divide myself, as it were, into two persons: and that I, the examiner and judge, represent a different character from that other I, the person whose conduct is examined into and judged of.

> The first is the Spectator whose sentiments with regard to my own conduct I endeavour to enter into.... The second is the Agent, the person whom I properly call myself. (Smith in Hoskin 1996: 155)

The formulation of the self as rational through a heuristic division into two (examiner and judge) makes 'reflexivity' possible, since there is a logical space between the 'I' (as a putative centre of consciousness) and the 'me' (what others identify as the 'I'). Hoskin (1996) uses the distinction to argue that our sense of being a discrete autonomous individual is learned though processes of social interaction, in which it is normal to become an object to oneself. As Hume argued, the way we become ethical is to consider how our actions are viewed by an 'impartial spectator' – an ethical touchstone of what 'ought' to be. This 'other', redefined as part of the self, produces a new form of rational self as split: a self that acts, and a self that examines those acts. As an accountable self, 'I' become moral through this process.

Conclusion

Beck and Beck-Gernsheim (1995) argue that having children is increasingly connected with hopes of being rooted and of life becoming meaningful, and with a 'claim to happiness' based on the close (and understood to be permanent) relationship with the child. Having a child is a meaningful experience, because it is an experience of the self:

> The desire for children [is] ego-related and connected with the present: parents want to ... get something for themselves from giving birth, nursing, raising and providing for their children.... Hope of discovering oneself through one's children is more widespread ... it is [typical] of a large number of parents that having children is no longer primarily understood as a service, a kind of devotion of social obligation. Instead it is admitted to be a way of life in which one pursues one's own interests (Beck and Beck-Gernsheim 1995: x).

Parenting is not merely about how adults react to children, then; it is also about how adults make statements about themselves (Furedi 2002: 107). In deciding how to dress, feed, put to sleep and transport their children, adults do not simply live their lives through children but, in part, develop their own identity through them.

Notes

1. These are not real addresses; rather, they reflect the type of email addresses it was common to see.
2. Buskens uses 'romantic' and 'rational-efficiency', terms I find somewhat problematic and replace with 'unstructured' and 'structured'.
3. More than two-thirds of working-age women with dependent children (68 per cent) were working in the second quarter of 2008. Sixty-seven per cent of women of working age (18–65) are employed in the UK (OECD).
4. Brazelton interviewed in 1988 on *The World of Ideas* by Bill Moyers. Cited in Eyer (1992: 4).
5. As Onora O'Neill remarked recently, at a *Guardian Forum* (2010) the idea of parenthood as a form of self-expression is now intimately tied up with developments in the world of Artificial Reproductive Technologies.

Chapter 2

INFANT FEEDING AND
INTENSIVE MOTHERHOOD

Charlotte: What has your experience of breastfeeding been like?

Sylvia [37, breastfeeding her 17- and 2-month-old daughters]: Very positive. Challenging at times but overall, incredibly rewarding, life-changing … enlightening. It has made me a better mother, lover, wife, sister, daughter.

This chapter explores the relationship between infant feeding, intensive mothering and maternal identity work. As a substance, breast milk 'seeps' – to use Carsten's phrase[1] – between the domains of the familial (in the sense that it creates relatedness) and the biomedical (in the sense that it is an object of scientific investigation). The chapter therefore opens by briefly outlining the physiological processes of breastfeeding before turning to consider recent policy directives and demographic patterns of infant feeding. Women in the perinatal period can expect to hear a strong 'breast is best' message from a range of governmental and nongovernmental agencies, although at the level of practice, women's experiences of receiving this message are highly variable (Lee 2007a, Battersby 2006).

Whilst supporting women in carrying out their infant-feeding decisions is clearly desirable, this chapter calls attention to the difference between support and advocacy, which generic 'pro-breastfeeding' policies often seem to conflate. In exploring the relationship between public ideologies and individual desires, is important to recognise that the fact that so many women 'want' to breastfeed, and to breastfeed for particular lengths of time, is an outcome of these very policies advocating breastfeeding as best. Yet the 'breast is best' message is a simplification, and a clumsy one at that: not only does it often overplay the benefits of breastfeeding, but it also eclipses many other aspects of the feeding relationship that mothers must also take into account. This has the potential to diminish choice, properly defined, and can have quite negative consequences. The chapter therefore closes with a look at infant feeding 'at the margins', discussing the experiences of women whose infants were formula-fed in the early months (Lee 2008; Murphy 1999, 2003) as a means of setting up a comparison with the attachment mothers focused on here. With infant feeding a critical element of maternal identity work, 'norms' surrounding maternal identity and feeding practices are contextualised.

Breastfeeding

'Try sucking the tip of your finger,' says Janet, at one of the monthly La Leche League meetings in North West London.[2] We all do. 'Can you feel how your tongue flattens the tip on to the roof of your mouth? And how your teeth touch it?' We chorus a yes through our fingertips. 'Now put your finger deeper into your mouth – to the second knuckle, and suck again. Can you feel the difference? The tongue is now elongated and massaging the whole length of your finger. The jaw isn't closed and hard, but open and more relaxed, isn't it? Your teeth and the finger are hardly touching either.'

Janet uses this demonstration to show the difference between a baby who is poorly latched on to the mother's nipple and one who is properly attached to her breast. Without being latched on properly, she explains, the likelihood is that a baby will not be able to draw out enough milk and, in turn, will not grow well. It is also likely that breastfeeding will be extremely painful for the mother. 'It's not called nipple-feeding, is it?' says Janet. 'Breastfeeding is what we want.' She uses the example to show how many common breastfeeding problems (sore nipples, blocked ducts, mastitis, failure to thrive, etc.) can often be prevented by basic knowledge of effective positioning.

As much as it is 'instinctual', then, breastfeeding is a technique of the body, like walking, swimming or having sex, that must be learned (Mauss 1973). Sadly, this information came too late for many of the women encountered during the course of this research. Over the course of fieldwork, numerous women reported that they had rarely held a baby, let alone seen one being breastfed, before giving birth to their own children. LLL can be credited with providing backup for a health-care system that leaves many women without adequate information about or support for breastfeeding. Warning that 'breast is best' without providing real means of achieving this puts many women in a terrible bind. I briefly explain the physiological process of breastfeeding here, based on information shared during fieldwork and additional reading.

Breasts are made up of a system of ducts, embedded in fatty tissue, supplied with blood, and connected by nerve endings. The process of 'lactogenesis' begins during pregnancy, creating milk. Within each of these ducts, many thousands of cells, called alveoli, manufacture milk by absorbing water, salts, sugar and fat from the blood (Small 1998: 187). There is little relation between breast size and the amount of milk a woman is able to produce. During pregnancy, higher levels of the hormones oestrogen and progesterone stimulate the alveoli to multiply in a 'branching' fashion within the breast. Although most women do not secrete milk until after the birth of their baby, a thick fluid called colostrum is produced and passed through the breasts from around the sixth month of pregnancy onwards. This fluid is high in protein, low in sugar and fat, and immunological.

The level of prolactin, a hormone in the mother's body associated with the regulation of lactation, amongst other things, drops following the birth of a baby but remains above pre-pregnancy rates, rising again when the newborn starts to suckle. At this point, nerve endings in the mother's nipple stimulate the release of more prolactin and another hormone, oxytocin. This encourages milk to flow down the branch-like structures to the area behind the mother's nipple, and eventually into the baby's mouth.

Milk is produced in the mother's breasts, but the infant is key to getting it from one body into the other. Infants typically have a 'rooting' reflex whereby they search for a nipple, and a sucking reflex when that nipple is in the mouth: the tongue pushes forward to squeeze the nipple against the top of the mouth and release milk (although a range of factors may inhibit this). Milk replaces colostrum in the first few days after birth (generally on the third day).

Milk production typically works on a supply-and-demand basis. Ideally, the more a baby drinks, the more the mother's body produces – so for as long as there is a demand, there will generally be a supply. As I discuss further below, however, these 'ideal' scenarios of the breastfeeding process are not always borne out in women's experiences.

The 'Scientific Case' for Breastfeeding

Milk is an evocative substance, particularly in British society, which attaches a high status to dairy products in the diet (Dupuis 2002).

Most images of milk are of cow's milk – thick, white liquid poured over cereal or made into cream, cheese or yoghurt. Thus a sense of revelation was an enduring feature of my fieldwork in LLL groups. Like many of the new mothers I met there, I was fascinated by the mechanisms of lactation and found it enlightening to learn so much about the capacities of the breast, and of breast milk. I remember it being said, to gasps of delight from the assembled group, that breast milk is an antiseptic whose topical application clears up a range of infections, including conjunctivitis (Pishva et al. 1998).[3]

Antibodies acquired via the mother's placenta circulate in the bloodstream at birth, but infants require contact with the outside world to build up their own immunological repertoire. Breast milk, which contains antibodies formulated by the mother in response to her environment, is one means of supporting the infant's immune system. Indeed, these immunological factors in breast milk are the primary reason breastfed infants suffer fewer gastrointestinal (GI) infections than their formula-fed counterparts (Victoria et al. 1987, Howie et al. 1990).

Today, studies suggesting links between breastfeeding and protection against Sudden Infant Death Syndrome (SIDS) (Bernshaw 1991) and between breast milk and reductions in the number of respiratory infections (Cunningham, Jelliffe and Jelliffe 1991; Goldman, 1993; Newman 1995, citing Slade and Schwartz 1987), later inflammatory bowel syndrome (Klement et al. 2005), diabetes (Sadauskaite-Kuehne et al. 2004), cancers (American Institute for Cancer Research 2008), asthma (Oddy et al. 2002), allergies (Chandra 1997; Marini et al. 1996) and ear infections (Bitoun 1994; Duncan et al. 1993) are widely cited in literature around infant feeding (this list comes from Small [1998: 196], an advocate of attachment parenting). UNICEF lists, in addition, reduced rates of pneumonia, urinary tract infections (Marild, Jodal and Hanson 1990) and necrotising enterocolitis (amongst premature babies) in breastfed infants (UNICEF, National Childbirth Trust and Save the Children 2007). LLL also notes (LLLI 2004: chap. 18 passim) that breastfed children have better jaw and eye development (Birch et al. 1993; Davis and Bell 1991) and are protected from obesity in later life (Gillman et al. 2001). Other studies suggest a link between breastfeeding and higher IQ in infants (Lucas et al. 1994; Mortensen et al. 2002; Rogan and Gladen 1993)[4] and enhanced maternal 'bonding' (Lavelli and Polli 1998; Sears 2003).[5] These claims, however, require some contextualisation, as I explore below.

The effects of breastfeeding on women's health are also widely promoted. Breastfeeding typically releases oxytocin, which can help the uterus pull back into shape after birth and stem any residual post-partum bleeding (American Academy of Pediatrics 1997). Breastfeeding, said to use between 500 and 1,000 calories a day, can use up some of the extra fat stored during pregnancy (although women do also need to eat slightly more to sustain this; see Dewey, Heinig and Nommsen 1993). As part of a wider reproductive package, breastfeeding (at sustained levels) may also have a contraceptive effect, as it can suppress ovulation (causing lactational amenorrhea; see Kennedy and Visness 1992). Women who breastfeed for longer periods are said to be at a lower risk of osteoporosis (Commings and Klineberg 1993) and breast and uterine cancers (Rosenblatt and WHO 1993; United Kingdom National Case-Control Study Group 1993) than those who do not breastfeed (UNICEF et al. 2007).

The Context of Infant Feeding, 1900–Present

From about 1900, infant feeding in Britain became an explicit state concern as part of broader government policies to combat infant mortality (Carter 1995: 41). Education about breastfeeding, coupled with the development of milk dispensaries that supplied hygienic equipment and 'pure milk' at reduced cost to mothers whose babies needed artificial milk, was the earliest state action targeting infant nutrition. By 1905, twelve such centres existed (Carter 1995: 44). Just thirty years later, during the Second World War, mothers received powdered milk subsidies, seen by this point to be an essential investment in the health of the nation.

The medicalisation of childbirth during the 1940s and 1950s, represented by the growth in hospital births from 15 per cent in 1927 to 66 per cent in 1958 (Carter 1995: 58), had a profound impact on feeding experiences. Women were increasingly subject to the routinisation requirements of the hospital, which were not conducive to breastfeeding. The medical profession did not advise women to formula feed per se, but the care they offered implicitly led women to do so. 'Although breastfeeding remained official policy, little attention was paid to it,' writes Carter (1995: 58). Relatively rapidly, women were having babies in institutional settings. This was in contrast to previous generations, whose extended families lived in closer proximity and whose children were born at home. Given that hospital staff were not provided with training in breastfeeding but were, however, trained in making bottles of formula (often subsidised by formula manufacturers), it is unsurprising that rates of breastfeeding fell in congruence with growing hospitalisation.

Tellingly, when the British National Health Service was established in 1948, over 75 per cent of British mothers initiated the breastfeeding of their infants (Rogers, Emmett and Golding 1997). By 1970, a generation later, there had been a marked decline to nearly half the former rate (Butler and Golding 1986). In the period from 1964 to 1974, formula feeding reached its peak in Britain. Most importantly, this established an understanding between mothers and health professionals that breastfeeding was 'natural' but required expert advice and intervention to be successful (i.e., it should be regimented). Thus both breast and bottle-feeding were subject to scientisation during this time.

As noted, Apple (1987), writing about the same period in the United States (between the late nineteenth and the mid-twentieth century), sees this as the time when mothers lost their central position in the experience of feeding and care. In the space of three generations, babies became bottle-fed under medical supervision rather than nursed at their mothers' breasts. This effectively allied formula manufacturers with physicians in a move that undermined women's ability to care for their babies. But Jacqueline Wolf (2001), again writing about the United States, points out that feminists have often overlooked how women themselves were key players in the decrease in breastfeeding and the routine use of formula milk. Rather than simply bowing to the will of medics who had an interest in appropriating childrearing from women, or to men who wanted women's bodies for their own sexual gratification, Wolf argues that women – particularly those who worked outside the home – welcomed the use of bottled milk. Formula milk was also welcomed by those who felt breastfeeding to be shameful, tied to notions of the breasts as sexualised, private parts of the body, writes Carter (1995) about the UK. Furthermore, not only did these methods promise to ease the stresses of dealing with infant care, but women believed the widely promoted idea that formula feeding was the optimal way of feeding infants. And as Apple put it in a recent talk, 'What mother would want to risk the health of her baby by not doing "The Best"?'[6]

Yet since the 1970s, the dominant turn has been to a discursive environment in which breastfeeding is validated as 'best' by a wide range of social actors – including breastfeeding campaign groups, medical authorities and the state (Lee 2007a, 2007b, 2008; Murphy 1999, 2003). The revival of interest in breastfeeding during the 1970s was demonstrated by more research being published on its health benefits. Carter points out that in the government's 1980 report, fewer doubts were expressed about breastfeeding's benefits than in

1943 (Carter 1995: 60). Today, the UK government, in line with the World Health Organization (WHO), advises exclusive breastfeeding for six months and continued breastfeeding, in conjunction with other foods, for up to two years or beyond (Department of Health [DH] 2005a).

UNICEF's Baby Friendly Initiative, a programme drawn up in 1992 and active in the UK since 1994, is currently endorsed as the gold standard of maternity care by the National Institute for Clinical Excellence and the Department of Health. Maternity facilities receive accreditation as 'Baby Friendly' by adopting the initiative's *10 Steps to Successful Breastfeeding*.[7] Baby Friendly accreditation requires having a written breastfeeding policy that is routinely communicated to all staff, training staff in how to implement this policy, informing all pregnant women about the benefits of breastfeeding and helping women initiate breastfeeding soon after birth (UNICEF 2005). Hospital staff must not provide infants with any food or drink other than breast milk, 'unless medically indicated'. Similarly, demonstrating how to formula feed a baby is to take place only upon a mother's specific request, and never in groups. Group demonstrations are reserved for information on how to breastfeed. If mothers do decide to use formula milk, they are to do so only 'after being fully informed of the benefits of exclusive breastfeeding and the risks of supplementary feeding' (UNICEF 2005). The programme has shown some success in raising the initiation rates of breastfeeding: a recent study showed that babies born in Baby Friendly hospitals were 28 per cent more likely to be breastfed at seven days than those born elsewhere (Broadfoot et al. 2005).

Infant Feeding and Policy

Women consider a huge range of factors when making decisions about how to feed their babies (Carter 1995; Lee 2007a, 2007b), but a mother's social class, age and educational level are all associated with (if not causal in) the incidence of breastfeeding. Analysis of national trends reveals a gradual increase in rates of breastfeeding since the low point in the 1970s. Between 1995 and 2005, for example, breastfeeding at birth[8] in the UK rose by 10 per cent, from 66 per cent to 76 per cent. When analysed by socio-economic classification, the highest incidence of breastfeeding babies aged 6 to 10 weeks in the UK was found among mothers from managerial and professional occupations, at 88 per cent. The lowest incidence of breastfeeding was found among mothers in routine and manual occupations and mothers who had never worked, both at 65 percent.

The 2005 Infant Feeding Survey (the most recent statistics available at the time of research, conducted by the government every five years) showed that 48 per cent of mothers in the UK were breastfeeding (exclusively or in combination) at 6 weeks, while 25 per cent were still breastfeeding at 6 months.[9] Yet by 6 months, the rates of exclusive breastfeeding (with no other fluid given to the baby) were negligible across the UK. The decrease is rapid: only 35 per cent of babies were being exclusively breastfed at 1 week, 21 per cent at 6 weeks, 7 per cent at 4 months and 3 per cent at 5 months. Early results from the 2010 survey indicate little change in these patterns (DH 2011).

These patterns of infant feeding are increasingly a target for policy intervention, with early feeding patterns presented as determining lifelong patterns of eating and health (cancers, coronary heart disease and obesity are highlighted in particular). Infant feeding has been a central part of health policy since the 1990s, with the Department of Health aiming to raise awareness about the benefits of breastfeeding – which are now taken as unequivocal – and to increase breastfeeding rates, especially in low-income groups (DH 2004a, 2004b, 2005a, 2005b, 2005c, cited in Lee and Bristow 2009). The mental and emotional health of mothers and babies is deemed to be improved by breastfeeding, and breastfeeding is increasingly associated with 'good parenting' as well as a driving belief that societal inequality (in terms of health outcomes) will decrease if more women breastfeed (Lee 2011).

An example of this is the Breastfeeding Manifesto Coalition, a grouping of diverse organisations (including LLL) who came together in 2006 to counter health inequalities across the UK through the promotion of breastfeeding.[10] Online, the manifesto states that the coalition is 'working to improve awareness of the health benefits of breastfeeding and its role in reducing health inequalities across the UK.... Evidence demonstrates that breastfeeding ... leads to significant health benefits for mothers, can counteract health inequalities, leaves no ecological footprint and saves money.' (Breastfeeding Manifesto Coalition 2007). The coalition points to an interesting relationship between the state and non-governmental organisations (NGOs). The manifesto, designed to lobby government ministers and calling for greater promotion of and support for breastfeeding, has been very well received. At its launch, then Minister for Public Health Caroline Flint endorsed its aims, and over 250 parliamentarians have now given their support to achieving its goals.

As Lee and Furedi (2005) rightly point out, the choices mothers make today as to how to feed their babies remain most likely to be narrated within this wider arena of debates about health, showing how, in the past few decades, the promotion of 'healthy living' has received enormous attention. The UK government understands health as something individuals should be enabled to choose, through educational programs facilitating alteration of their behaviour (*Choosing Health* was the name of one DH white paper in 2004 [Department of Health 2004b]). As Fitzpatrick argues, '"Health" has come to operate as a "secular moral framework" for society, emphasising individual responsibility and … compliance with the appropriate medically sanctioned standard of behaviour" (Fitzpatrick 2004: 70). As Peterson and Lupton (1996) note about the 'New Public Health', the approach focuses on behaviour modification, since people's behaviour is considered the primary reason for ill health (as opposed to social or material conditions). Healthy lifestyles become an expression of engagement with a particular political regime and a form of self-expression for the responsible citizen – a responsibility heightened in the case of mothers charged with maintaining the health of their children. Policies that demand people conform to government norms can be justified by the rhetoric of 'supporting' people in making 'informed choices', and 'support' extended to those considered in need of help, whether they want it or not: 'Support rarely means assisting people to improve what they are already struggling to do. In practice, it means placing pressure on people to adopt a course of action favoured by the government. "Promote health by influencing people's attitudes to the choices they make", is how one government strategy document puts it' (Furedi 2005).

Part of the new health paradigm is an injunction to the individual to minimise risks from so-called 'bad' foods (and arguably to individualise wider social patterns). This carries particular moral baggage for mothers: 'The health of children in particular has been identified as a potent site for risk consciousness in this regard because of their presumed innocence and vulnerability … and for this reason, it has been argued that, because mothers have a particular responsibility for feeding children, the moralisation of eating intersects with the social construction of motherhood' (Lee 2007b; see also Lupton 1996). In an era of intensive motherhood, the injunction that mothers 'maximise' the wellbeing of their children is primarily narrated in the language of risk and health. Today, mothers who do not breastfeed are no longer presented as ignorant or careless (Carter 1995), but as needing more 'support'. As Murphy notes, however, this tends to be in the form of verbal encouragement rather than increased material resources (which would allow mothers time to rest, run the home or look after other children as well as manage the requirements of exclusive breastfeeding) (Blum 1999; Murphy 2003).

Choosing to Breastfeed: Informed Choice?

Where breastfeeding is the officially endorsed method of infant feeding, enacting an 'informed choice' arguably means choosing to breastfeed.[11] Yet the scientific case in favour of breastfeeding is less clear-cut than the policy literature might suggest. For example, whilst there is a real difference in the number of GI infections in breastfed and formula-fed children, it is perhaps a smaller one than might be assumed: one of the most widely respected studies of this in the developed world indicated that for every twenty-five breast-fed babies there would be one fewer GI infection in the first year (Kramer 2001). It should also be noted that – in the UK, at least – children who are breastfed are more likely to be in close proximity to their mothers, and therefore less exposed to pathogens, than children in, for example, day care, who are more likely to be formula-fed, which may skew these results further.

A table reproduced from Hoddinott, Tappin and Wright (2008) as Appendix 1 summarises the differential outcomes and comments on the reliability of the data used in making the various claims around breastfeeding. This table is useful because it points to the gap that exists between the reliability of much of the 'scientific case' for breastfeeding and the arguments made by many breastfeeding advocates. Indeed, these claims require some serious interrogation, and it is worth noting that numerous studies have *not* shown a link between breast milk consumption and the outcomes above.

The sociologist Joan Wolf notes that whilst numerous studies find that the average breastfed baby *is* healthier than the average formula-fed baby, there is no compelling evidence that breastfeeding *causes* better health (2011). Correlation, as she says, does not equal causation, as multiple factors need to be taken into account. Quite problematically, many of the studies that show benefits of breastfeeding fail to adjust for the socio-economic variables that have been shown to influence health (see Law 2000), and ultimately, no comparative trial can control for an individual mother's decision to breastfeed or not, regardless of whether class is controlled for. A mother's decision to breastfeed represents more than her social class; it reflects a certain orientation towards parenting that itself might be correlated with certain outcomes in terms of IQ or health.

There is often a slippage, too, in the presentation of the scientific case for breastfeeding – breastfeeding is a practice, whilst breast milk is a substance (Hausman 2003: 19). Knaak (2006) also notes that pro-breastfeeding discourse generally discusses the relative mortality and morbidity risks of formula feeding by referring to global statistics, which include data from countries that are incomparable, in terms of access to clean water and sanitation, to either North America or the UK. She comments that the differential outcomes between formula-fed and breastfed babies are 'on balance, considerably less pronounced than the [pro-breastfeeding] discourse portrays'.[12]

Wolf therefore argues that the evidence around breastfeeding is incomplete, methodologically problematic and often inconclusive (see her 2011 *Is Breast Best?* for a full dissection of these claims). In Chapter 7, I discuss further some of the issues around scientisation, knowledge claims and policymaking. Certainly, if the science is less conclusive than is currently presented, this poses some interesting questions around 'informed choice' and 'evidence-based policy'.

Yet – as is true of much popular reporting of science – this uncertainty and ambiguity is screened out of literature parents can expect to encounter when working out how to feed their children. On the basis of her study of Dr Spock's manual (and the several editions published between 1946 and 1998), Knaak (2005) shows how the advice mothers receive about infant feeding has gradually become more and more child-centred, in accordance with an intensive motherhood framework. (The manual itself has become ever longer in accordance with the rise of expertise and the increased amount of information available.) Whereas forty years ago, for example, both breastfeeding and formula feeding were presented as options with pros and cons for mother and baby, now formula milk is presented as best avoided. 'Choice in infant feeding has become constrained discursively to the point where it has become more directive than a choice ... [and] the very existence of choice in infant feeding [between the two options] has become suspect' (Knaak 2005: 212). In this environment, a positive value is associated with breastfeeding – and by extension, a negative one with the choice to formula feed. Kate, an LLL leader, gives a good example of this:

> Kate [*in her late 30s, breastfeeding her 5-year-old daughter*]: According to the WHO, formula feeding isn't even second best, it is fourth option after actually feeding at the breast, feeding your baby by expressing

your own milk, or feeding your baby with the milk of another woman ... but people don't know that, and there is a perception that it is almost as good, or just as good, and therefore it is *just* a lifestyle choice ... [it shouldn't be] 'Breastfed babies have a decreased risk' of getting asthma or whatever ... [it] should be 'Breastfed babies have the normal risk for your species, and formula-fed children have a higher risk'. All things being equal ... there is something perfectly designed for your baby, for your species that will make sure its brain develops correctly. Cow's milk has all the things for a *calf's* muscle development. Breast milk has all the immunologically balanced stuff, and is nutritionally ideal ... even when they know what things are in breast milk, they don't know what quantities to put into formula milk, because the things in breast milk are perfectly bioavailable, balanced.... The idea of an optional extra as if it doesn't matter if you do or if you didn't ... doesn't do anyone any favours.

Formula milk was referred to as 'junk food' in an article in *The Ecologist* (Thomas 2006), alongside claims that this early diet of 'convenience food' was the cause of death and illness in children. Some advocates even propose that formula packages should carry warning labels and be kept locked up, to be given out only on medical prescription (LLL meeting observation).

From Preference to Obligation

In *Being Good*, the philosopher Blackburn (2001) uses the example of the abortion debate in the United States to talk about how social problems get moralised, 'becoming not just a question of sympathy or concern, which admit of gradations, but of who has *rights*, or what *justice* requires, or what our *duty* is; it is a question of what is *permissible* and what is *wrong*.' He notes that these are called 'deontological' notions, after the Greek *deontos*, meaning duty. 'They have a coercive edge. They take us beyond what we admire, or regret, or prefer, or even what we want other people to prefer. They take us to thoughts about what is *due*. They take us to demands' (Blackburn 2001: 61).

In their article 'Rules for Feeding Babies', Lee and Bristow (2009) look at the relationship between infant feeding and state regulation (see also Murphy 1999). They note that whether a woman breastfeeds, whilst not (yet) a question of law, is nevertheless a 'juridical' domain, featuring a plethora of campaigns to encourage women to breastfeed with related messages about what women should and should not do (Lee and Bristow 2009). The authors note that so far, no country has imposed a law that forces women to breastfeed (though in fact, a Prussian law of 1794 went so far as to require that healthy women nurse their own babies [Schiebinger 1993: 41]). Yet many breastfeeding advocates, and many of the attachment mothers with whom I worked, argue for a child's 'right to be breastfed'. Amelia, very active in the breastfeeding community, said:

> *Amelia [33, breastfeeding her almost-3-year-old son]*: For me it [breastfeeding] borders on being a basic human right. And the fewer people that do it, the fewer people that think it is normal the more the rights of mums to breastfeed is going to be curtailed.

As Lee and Bristow note, those who advocate the 'right' to be breastfed, or even the right to breastfeed, tend to frame their case in a specific way:

> First, they represent the mother as also in need of new rights (rather than duties). 'Infants have a human right to be breastfed, and women have the right to be empowered to fulfil this duty,' claims one pro-breastfeeding campaigner (Mahabal 2004). The legal means advocated through which the 'empowerment of women' to give them the 'right to breastfeed' is to be brought about are usually measures that purport to 'protect' women from damaging influences. These are primarily laws to restrict advertising of formula milk, and to enable breastfeeding in public places. (Lee and Bristow 2009: 83)

In the UK, both types of law have been enacted – the marketing of formula milks for infants is tightly regulated, and the Right to Breastfeed Act was effectively passed in April 2010 as part of the Equalities Act (Department for Communities and Local Government, Commons Leader 2009).[13] Attention is drawn to this, not to dispute the need for these laws – since it is rather paradoxical that under a government that encourages breastfeeding so strongly, it may be legal for someone to stop a woman doing so in public – but rather to show the legal spaces that have opened up around maternal behaviour, the almost exclusive focus on health benefits to the child and the antagonistic language in which it is framed.

A Bottle-Feeding Culture?

Yet whilst breastfeeding is validated as best in the *discursive* environment, it would be wrong to say that breastfeeding is unambiguously promoted and supported. Many women I met told me of health professionals who were sceptical about the benefits of breastfeeding and, they felt, unsupportive of the practice. At a wider cultural level, in the course of perinatal care, women can expect to hear the 'breast is best' message, yet many scholars, as well as breastfeeding advocates – like Caroline, cited in the introduction – have claimed that that we actually live in what is termed a 'bottle-feeding culture' where breastfeeding is frequently undermined (Scott 2003).

Four factors are normally cited as contributing to the production of a bottle-feeding culture: media; sexual aesthetics; the influence of formula milk manufacturers; and limited, inflexible working arrangements that are said to create a negative public perception of breastfeeding and thereby implicitly sustain a bottle-feeding culture (Reeve 1997).

Women appearing in soap operas, or in advertisements for consumer goods not explicitly linked to infant feeding, typically appear bottle-feeding their infants, for example. The baby bottle is a symbol for the baby changing room in many public locations, and many maternity cards, dolls and illustrations of babies come accompanied by bottles (although this is starting to change under pressure from lobby groups, and recently a 'breast milk baby' doll was released in the US [2011]).

Certainly, women can face opposition to their breastfeeding by members of the public – being asked to 'cover up' on public transport, or to leave restaurants and shops, and several women reported this to me during fieldwork (although many others reported receiving positive comments too). During the time of research, 'nurse-ins', or breastfeeding flash mobs, were a common response to this sort of criticism, and I explore this in Chapter 5 as a form of activism.

In terms of sexual and aesthetic factors, women are clearly in a difficult position. They are advised that breastfeeding is natural and normal and 'nothing to be ashamed of', yet at the same time, it is to be managed discreetly. Many women struggle with this paradox, particularly with reference to their sexuality and in their relationships with partners who may be unsupportive of their desire to breastfeed (Earle 2002 Marshall, Godfrey and Renfrew 2007; Schmidt 2008; Scott 2003). As Carter notes, it is not helpful to simply assert that breasts are not really sexual, because they have been coded as sexual in a way that is deeply ingrained throughout our culture (Carter 1995: 157). Mothers are typically obliged to manage the 'gaze' of others by keeping their breasts covered whilst feeding – not the easiest of tasks. And indeed, this is reflected in the advice women receive as to the sorts of clothes they should wear. La Leche League counsels women to wear a shawl to nurse discreetly, though it also advocates 'feeding with pride'. Many women encountered during fieldwork were involved in public displays of breastfeeding at 'nurse-ins', though others felt that this was 'too militant' and not a way to encourage women to breastfeed. A more recent campaign from the organisation Best Beginnings, the charity behind the *Breastfeeding Manifesto,* tries to address and promote the paradox with a poster showing a naked women's torso with a baby's hand on one breast and a partner's hand on the other (Figure 2.1). The tag line reads, 'Bond with your baby, bond with your man'.

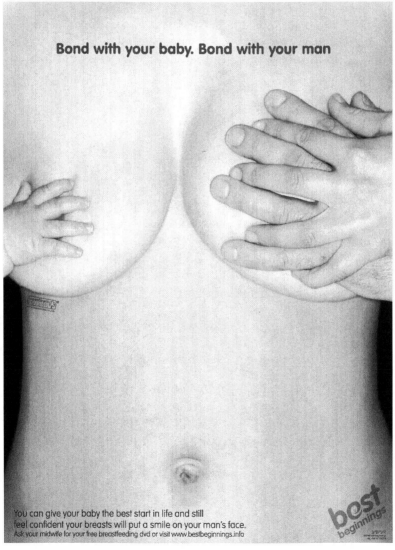

FIGURE 2.1. Best Beginnings poster, 'Bond with your baby, bond with your man', 2008, reproduced with permission of Best Beginnings

The place of formula milk manufacturers is also routinely called into in these debates. In 1995 a law was introduced in the UK to ban the marketing of formula milks to parents. It was argued that such marketing undermined breastfeeding and negatively affected breastfeeding rates (Dyson et al. 2006; Renfrew et al. 2005). The law implemented parts of the WHO's *International Code of Marketing of Breastmilk Substitutes*, drawn up in the aftermath of the Nestlé affair of the 1970s (see Palmer [1993] and Raphael and Davis [1985] for contrasting accounts of this).[14] Since the 1995 law, which set out to ban advertising of infant formula to parents (i.e., formula for children under 6 months old), companies have developed 'follow-on' formulas for older babies, designed to look identical to infant formulas, as a means of advertising their brand to parents. Various lobby groups and NGOs have unsuccessfully attempted to close this loophole (UNICEF et al. 2007).[15]

I do not dwell on these dilemmas here, but the advertising issue points to some interesting tensions within feminist discourses around infant feeding, most notably around choice. A clear link between the advertising of follow-on milks and parents' decisions has never actually been proven (Food Standards Agency 2009): What this argument screens out, then, is women's desire (or otherwise) to fulfil these policy recommendations (i.e., it is assumed women want to breastfeed, but the advertising sways them from this). Yet as noted earlier, even statistics on women's desire to breastfeed, which are taken to endorse these measures to limit advertising under the guise of 'protecting' mothers, must be viewed in light of the cultural context that validates breastfeeding as the 'best' way of feeding a baby (thus, asking a woman who is now formula feeding whether she 'wanted to breastfeed for longer' is not a morally neutral question).

A final point that is brought to bear in these debates is that limited leave and lack of flexible work make combining breastfeeding and working difficult for mothers, but this is more typical in the US, where six weeks' leave is standard (see Hausman 2003). In the UK, the story is a little different. In 2008 (just after the time of data collection), maternity leave was extended from six months to one year (although this is nowhere near fully paid, Directgov 2011),[16] and the government has been working to improve the situation for working mothers. Of course, not all mothers are able to take advantage of these changes, and socio-economic ability to make these 'choices' is reflected in statistics that show a correlation between breastfeeding and women of means and education.

Infant Feeding and Maternal Identity

Women clearly sit at the juncture of multiple and competing messages around infant feeding. Yet the idea that there is a 'moral context' for infant feeding is upheld by virtually all studies about maternal experience. Miller, Bonas and Dixon-Woods suggest that a dominant theme that emerges from the qualitative literature is that mothers often experience infant feeding as a moral problem, and that infant feeding decisions and practices are experienced as a measure of motherhood: 'The literature suggests that perceived societal and peer pressure, the expectations of health professionals, and feelings of guilt and concern over the need to be a 'good' mother profoundly shape not only the decisions and practices of women but also the accounts they offer of these.' (2007: 216).

This is echoed in work by the midwives Schmeid, Sheehan and Barclay on the accounts of women in Australia who choose to breastfeed their babies:

> The women in our studies believed that there was something 'special' about breast feeding [*sic*] and that they 'persevered' with breast feeding using extraordinary personal resources or resilience in their effort to create breast feeding as a connected, intimate and pleasurable activity. This commitment to, and perseverance with breast feeding, we believe is constructed within the current public rhetoric of 'breast is best', the spurious link between breast feeding and being a 'good' mother, and contemporary western concerns for rational, autonomous behaviour, control over the body and personal achievement. (Schmeid et al. 2001: 48)

The authors understand women's accounts as evidence of a desire to not only ensure what was best for the baby but create a particular identity as a mother. They were therefore concerned, as midwives, about the 'intensity of commitment, and almost religious fervour that some of these women conferred on their breastfeeding experience' (Schmeid et al. 2001: 48). That women would fashion their identities as mothers through how they fed their babies was both understandable and a cause for concern:

> We are concerned at the frequency of problems and the amount of distress and disruption that a breakdown of this desired breast feeding relationship may cause ... and speculate about the possibility that midwives and other health workers unwittingly contribute to this distress by somehow conveying that it is necessary to persevere with breast feeding through, for example, excruciating pain, to be a 'good' mother. (Schmeid et al. 2001: 48)

The intense commitment to breastfeeding, Schmeid et al. argue, is constructed within both popular and professional discourses that promote it as a symbol of good or successful mothering and a source of personal achievement. To go beyond what is considered reasonable becomes salient within the context of intensive mothering: the transformation of breastfeeding from a means of feeding a baby to a skill to be achieved leaves women who do not breastfeed open to the charge of failure. In this instance, breastfeeding has become a moral imperative.

Lee (2007a, 2007b, 2008) has written about her work with British mothers who use formula milk in the early months of their child's life. In a culture where 'breast is best,' her work addresses the moral work a woman has to undertake if, as Elizabeth Murphy puts it, she is to respond to the charge of being 'a 'poor mother' who places her own needs, preferences and convenience above her baby's welfare' (Murphy 1999: 187–188). The moralisation of infant feeding in a child-centred culture means women's choices intersect with maternal identity in an unprecedented way, she argues. Lee quotes one mother who says:

> They all got their boobs out, and then I got the bottle out ... then it was like a competition with the mums, about who had suffered most! You know, 'Oh well, you just have to suffer with it if you want the best for your baby'. So I was like 'you don't even know anything about me, and of course I want the best for my baby too'. (Lee 2007a: 1085)

Murphy (1999) notes that whether women breastfeed or formula feed, the link between breastfeeding, 'informed choice' and (good) motherhood is something to which *all* women must respond (see also Pain, Bailey and Mowl 2001). Being informed and reflexive becomes a moral injunction for (responsible) mothers, yet it is this very reflexivity that lays women open to the charge of deviancy:

> Assessments of maternal deviance rest, not upon whether the rules have been broken, but upon a judgement of the mother's agency in doing so. The moral mother is not simply one who follows the rules. Rather she is one who follows the rules *knowingly*. Conversely the deviant mother is not simply one who breaks the rules. Rather her deviance rests upon a [notion] ... that she breaks the rules *knowingly*. (Murphy 1999: 188)

Mothers in Murphy's study faced what she refers to as 'interactional challenges' (Murphy 1999: 187). They felt a need to justify why they were doing something they perceived as 'wrong' (see also Stapleton, Fielder and Kirkham 2008). Typically, they had used formula milk to address quite pragmatic issues, such as fatigue, a need to return to work, a wish to share feeding with another person or a dislike of the demands of breastfeeding, not to mention the pain that can be associated with positioning the baby on the breast. Yet they frequently felt defensive, angry, guilty and anxious at having to respond to criticism.

As Lee and Bristow (2009) comment, it is interesting that women who use formula milk feel that they are 'breaking the rules', as statistics show they are in the vast majority. The 2005 Infant Feeding Survey shows that by the time an infant is 6 weeks old, 79 per cent of mothers are not breastfeeding exclusively – meaning that at this point a majority of women are feeding their baby with some amount of formula milk. This leaves women to deal with what Murphy (1999) refers to as a feeling of 'moral jeopardy' – although this is a feeling that clearly diminishes as the child ages. Mothers who do not breastfeed in the early months must engage in 'identity work' to create themselves as moral citizens, in the face of 'deviance'. They do this, however, from within the comfort of a statistical, arguably cultural, norm of formula feeding.

I take up these findings and use them to 'think with' my own research with mothers who breastfeed for extended periods of time, or 'to full term', to explore how the moralisation of feeding affects women at the other end of the spectrum. The WHO (2003) states that breastfeeding in developed countries should continue 'for up to 2 years, or beyond' in conjunction with other foods, but the number of women who actually do this is very limited in the UK (in fact, statistics do not even exist for numbers of women breastfeeding beyond a year). Mothers who decide to breastfeed for 'long' periods of time therefore drift into a grey area, in the eyes of the state. These mothers must also undertake identity work – this time characterised by establishing themselves as 'non-conventional' but legitimate within the social context. Whilst they have the ideological backing of policy and an endorsement of their intensive mothering, in practice they are at the margins and can face sharp objections to their feeding practices. This is a self-justifying form of identity work, as opposed to the defensive work undertaken by formula-feeding mothers. Though the distinction between the two is porous, both discourses support and shape the 'breast is best' ideology. In embodying 'extremes' on the spectrum of infant feeding, both sets of women amplify issues around maternal identity, intensive motherhood and infant feeding.

Notes

1. J. Carsten, CUSAS Annual Lecture, Cambridge, 28 May 2009. Like blood, breast milk is a substance that translates across multiple domains.
2. Group name has been changed. This account is reproduced from notes.
3. As one reader notes, it is curious that here scientific claims and superstition often seem to be collapsed, presenting breast milk as having magical properties that can ward off all manner of evils.
4. But see Jain, Concato and Leventhal (2002) for a more critical look.
5. But see discussion below and especially Eyer (1992).
6. Advice to Mothers Conference, University of Warwick, June 2008.
7. In 2007 there were 51 fully accredited Baby Friendly maternity units across the UK, and a further 74 that had gone part way to accreditation by gaining a Certificate of Commitment. In 2011, 60 maternity facilities had full accreditation.
8. These figures should be read cautiously; breastfeeding at birth or 'initiation' means the baby has been put to the breast once.
9. Mothers may be breastfeeding exclusively (with no other substance given to the baby), breastfeeding in combination with formula milk, or formula feeding exclusively. In addition, many women express their breast milk to be used either in combination with formula feeding, or as a means of managing 'exclusive breastfeeding' (the provision of breast milk alone). I discuss expression in Chapter 9.
10. The Breastfeeding Manifesto Coalition counts among its members pro-breastfeeding advocacy groups, environmentalist groups, health professionals' organisations and other NGOs. At the time of writing the membership is listed as Amicus the Union, Association of Breastfeeding Mothers, Baby Feeding Law Group, Baby Milk Action, Best Beginnings, Biological Nurturing, Birthlight, BLISS, Bosom Buddies, Breastfeeding Network, Childfriendly Places, Community Practitioners' and Health Visitors' Association, Friends of the Earth, Independent Midwives Association, La Leche League Great Britain, Little Angels, Midwife Information and Resource Service, National Childbirth Trust, National Obesity Forum, Royal College of General Practitioners, Royal College of Midwives, Royal College of Nursing, Save the Children, Baby Café Charitable Trust, British Dietetic Association, Food Commission, Mother and Infant Research Unit, Royal College of General Practitioners, Royal College of Paediatrics and Child Health, United Kingdom Association for Milk Banking, UNICEF UK, UNISON, WOMB, Women's Environmental Network.
11. It is notable that breastfeeding is promoted under the auspices of UNICEF – i.e., the fund for children, as opposed to UNIFEM, the fund for women. Again, this is congruent with a wider intensive mothering framework endorsing child-centred care. Vanessa Maher also recognises the eclipsing of the mother here (Maher 1992: 157).

12. She refers to the paper 'Report of the Task Force on the Assessment of the Scientific Evidence Relating to Infant-Feeding Practices and Infant Health' (American Academy of Pediatrics 1984).

13. The bill generated protest from the breastfeeding community by stipulating a six-month limit. Many felt this would jeopardise women who breastfeed beyond that point in public (as also endorsed by the government). The debates continue.

14. In 1979 WHO/UNICEF hosted an international meeting on infant and young child feeding, following the widespread awareness of Nestlé's unethical marketing of formula milks in the developing world. The meeting, which included representatives of governments, health organisations, companies and campaigning groups, called for the development of an international code of marketing, as well as action on other fronts to improve infant and young child feeding practices. The International Baby Food Action Network (IBFAN) was formed by six of the campaigning groups at the meeting. The international code was drawn up in 1981 and passed by resolution in the European Parliament. It has still not been implemented as law in its entirety in the UK. The local branch of IBFAN in the UK, Baby Milk Action (BMA), monitors manufacturers' activities and campaigns for the code to be implemented as law. (Information from BMA website.) Many of the women I met in LLL also had ties to BMA or local organisations dedicated to monitoring advertising of formula milks.

15. I was actually involved in the writing of this report, working at the time as an intern at UNICEF in addition to continuing my PhD research. I now find much of the evidence and argument put forward problematic.

16. Statutory maternity leave now lasts 52 weeks (it was for 26 weeks at the time of research). Working women (full or part-time) are entitled to receive statutory maternity pay for up to 39 weeks of the leave (some may have additional packages from their employer). Different regulations apply for freelance workers or the self-employed. Statutory maternity pay is paid at 90 per cent of the average gross weekly earnings with no upper limit for the first six weeks; for the remaining 33 weeks it is paid at either the standard rate of £117.18 or 90 per cent of average gross weekly earnings (if this 90 per cent rate is less than the standard rate). Furthermore, couples are now able to 'split' parental leave on a six- and six-month basis through a system of transferable maternity leave, although statutory paternity leave was 2 weeks at the time of research.

Part II

La Leche League

Chapter 3

CONTEXTUALISING 'FULL-TERM' BREASTFEEDING

La Leche League

By 1956 in the United States, the rate of breastfeeding initiation amongst new mothers had dropped to an all-time low of 20 per cent (Cahill 2001). At a picnic of the lay Catholic Christian Family Movement in the Chicago suburbs that same year, two mothers nursed their babies under the shade of a tree, lamenting this fact. On hearing passing women comment that they wished they had been able to nurse their own babies, the two resolved, with five other mothers, to found La Leche League to support women who wanted to breastfeed (see Ward 2000 for a fuller look at the Catholic influence on LLL).

The name – pronounced 'lay-chey' – comes from a shrine in Florida to 'Nuestra Señora de La Leche y Buen Parto' (translated as 'Our lady of plentiful milk and good delivery') and was suggested at a time when 'breastfeeding' could not be used in public without 'offending sensibilities' (Cahill 2001: 31). At the first gathering of the group, in one of the founders' homes, the assembled mothers discussed a *Reader's Digest* article on the merits of breastfeeding. This set the precedent for an organisation devoted to giving 'information, education and support' to breastfeeding women. The La Leche League International (LLLI) by-laws state:

> The purpose of LLLI is charitable, educational and for the promotion of health: To help the mother learn to breastfeed her baby; To encour-

age good mothering through breastfeeding; To promote a better understanding of breastfeeding and related subjects. (LLLI Bylaws, 2004,
Article II, Section 1. General Purpose)

Over a period of months, the group put together its philosophy, perhaps most simply explained though the original tag line 'good mothering through breastfeeding' (later dropping the 'good' to be simply
'mothering through breastfeeding'). The league does not advocate
breastfeeding merely because of the nutritional benefits of mother's
milk, but is committed to certain views on motherhood, childrearing
and family life, of which (extended) breastfeeding forms a central
part (Gorham and Andrews 1990: 243). As a league, a purposeful
network, LLL was both a support group and an activist organisation
that played a major role in the revival of breastfeeding in the United
States and across the world.

Today, the organisation, called La Leche League International
(rather than just La Leche League) since 1964, reaches over 200,000
people every month in more than sixty-four countries through its
trained volunteers, whether in face-to-face monthly meetings, over
the telephone or via the Internet. Leaders, who run the groups, edit
(and in some cases write) the publications, and answer the telephones,
must have breastfed for at least one year and demonstrated a comprehensive knowledge of, and ability to live out, the LLL philosophy.

LLLI is a charity largely funded through donations and subscrip-
tions (though in some countries it receives state funding). It distin-
guishes itself as the sole global organisation devoted to the support
of breastfeeding mothers and works in an advisory role to the WHO
and UNICEF as a charitable NGO. The group is renowned worldwide as the foremost authority on breastfeeding. The first edition of
the group's manual *The Womanly Art of Breastfeeding* (1958) was little
more than a hand-typed pamphlet. Now in its seventh edition, it
spans nearly 500 pages and is available in twenty-seven languages.
This reveals, and indeed has shaped, the public appetite for information and support for breastfeeding. The group publishes magazines
for its leaders, members and interested health professionals, detail-
ing the latest research into breastfeeding. One of the more interesting developments in recent years has been the initiation of peer
counsellor programmes that target mothers in deprived communities that typically offer less support for breastfeeding women.

La Leche League was not the entire scope of the research into
infant feeding, which also included visiting around ten 'Baby Cafés'
established in London as part of a scheme to provide support for

breastfeeding women in disadvantaged communities. I also volunteered in a postnatal ward of a central London hospital over several months,[1] helping with its breastfeeding drop-in support service, and visited a Paris maternity hospital. I was also present at several Breastfeeding Manifesto Coalition meetings in London. These settings, in which alternative normalities of motherhood were expressed, were an important part of putting the practice of 'full-term' breastfeeding into a broader context.

Research Sample

I attended the monthly meetings of all LLL London and LLL Paris groups (at the time there were ten and eight groups respectively[2]) as a participant-observer over the course of eight months in London and four months in Paris during 2006–07, also going to any family days, couple or toddler meetings, conferences and leader workshops. Although there exists a 'mothers only' rule, students (typically of midwifery or medicine) are welcomed. I was granted access on this basis, having spoken with the Chair of the Council of Directors in each country, shown an 'information sheet', and offered a recommendation letter from my department.

LLL groups run on a four-month cycle, identical the world over. They address the benefits of breastfeeding, the family and the breastfed baby, the art of breastfeeding and avoiding difficulties, and nutrition and weaning. These are all explored in more depth in LLL publications. The meetings, generally held in a member's home, typically had between five and twenty mothers in attendance, with children ranging from newborn to 7 years old (the majority in the younger half of this spectrum). A leader would open the discussion before asking the women present to introduce themselves and their children, and raise any comments or concerns. The degree to which the meeting stuck to the specific 'meeting topic' depended wholly on the women present – some meetings were opened up immediately for 'burning questions', rather than being discussion-led.

After I had been attending a group for some time, I asked mothers there if they would be interested in talking to me more formally. Fewer than 900 members of La Leche League Great Britain (LLLGB) were 'paid-up' at the time of research, although nearly 8,000 women attended meetings in 2007, according to the 2008 report (LLLI 2008. This is compared with 2,500 paying members in France; statistics about the numbers of users were not available.)

Thus I did not make a distinction between those who were paid-up 'members' of LLL and those who were simply 'attendees' (one does not need to be a member to attend meetings, though many mothers do sign up to support their local group if they come regularly). All but one of those whom I approached agreed, and I thereby interviewed 26 mothers and 13 LLL leaders about their philosophy of parenting and experiences of breastfeeding. With permission, these interviews were recorded, transcribed and coded.

I interviewed women at a convenient time and place, generally in their own homes, typically for between 45 and 90 minutes. In these discussions, I was allowed to go beyond immediate horizons I encountered in the meetings – a particularly important opportunity for a researcher of a topic like motherhood. Since motherhood is a time of performance – both in the sense that through reflexivity, women act in deliberated ways with their children, and that they also do this consciously for an audience of peers – the meetings were not always spaces of easy speech. Indeed, a formal LLL system was in place, designed to keep the subject of the meeting on breastfeeding itself. Interviews were therefore a time for women to speak openly about those parts of the philosophy they endorsed, rejected or otherwise.

I also conducted an email survey, drawn up on the basis of the findings of the interviews, with 25 women in London and 23 in Paris. This survey offered a 'comparative tool' to facilitate a cross-cultural case study in Paris, as well as complementary data to ascertain a fuller demographic profile of my interviewees. The survey explored women's feeding decisions, asking if they felt under pressure to conform to certain social norms, and how their feeding decisions had affected the rest of their lives (e.g., relationships with friends, family or health professionals). It also asked women to expand more generally on their parenting experiences to talk about the difference between perceptions and experiences of parenting and how they differed from perceptions and experiences of motherhood. Writing being itself a reflexive practice, many of the comments women made on their questionnaires were highly informative. I suggest that this sort of small-scale survey data can be used to support more traditionally ethnographic findings, to the extent that the researcher has had the opportunity to spend periods of time with the people she intends to write about.

Whilst I present demographic results from the entire sample of women within LLL, in each country there are a few that I refer to as attachment mothers. These women practise an attachment parenting philosophy in addition to being members of LLL. That is, they typically breastfeed their children 'to full term'. The definition of full-term breastfeeding, following LLL convention, is taken to be breastfeeding beyond one year here (appreciating that one can feed 'to term' long after this point). LLL considers infants who self-wean after less than a year to be on a 'nursing strike' and suggests steps to interest them in breastfeeding again. Children who stop beyond the one-year mark are considered self-weaning, which is ideal. (This points to the cultural construction of so-called natural practices.) These attachment mothers also typically co-sleep and 'wear' their children, also opting for 'natural' alternatives to mainstream patterns of health care, food consumption, travel, clothing and so forth. Not all women undertake all of these elements with the same intensity, but there is certainly correlation around these sets of values. My classification is based on statistics and responses derived from the questionnaire – that is, from women breastfeeding their children beyond a year – as well as my own observations at group meetings and interviews.

In some cases, women who breastfed beyond a year were not classified as 'attachment' because they did not also ascribe to other elements of the attachment parenting philosophy. Similarly, some women had not yet breastfed beyond a year but definitely intended to, in line with attachment parenting philosophy. They are included in my definition of attachment mothers, and I draw on their accounts where relevant (i.e., not necessarily in reference to breastfeeding older children).

In the UK, the attachment mothers comprised approximately three quarters of the women I interviewed (16/22) and just over half (14/25) of the women who answered the questionnaire. In France, 3 of the 4 women interviewed were classified as attachment mothers, as were 7 out of 19 women who answered the questionnaire. All four of the women questioned in the anglophone group in Paris would also be classified as attachment mothers. Coding leaders as attachment or otherwise was more problematic, especially when their children were already grown or they had joined LLL in the days before 'attachment parenting' was so well known as a concept. Typically, older leaders did not call themselves attachment parents, whilst younger ones frequently demonstrated competence in and knowledge of many of the values and practices.

The Parisian case study is discussed separately in Chapter 9; from here, comments pertain only to the London sample.

Demographic Profile: Who Comes to LLL Meetings?

The twenty-five UK women who filled out questionnaires ranged between 23 and 47 years of age, the median age being 35.[3] The average age for having a first baby at the time of research in the UK was 29 (National Statistics Online 2008), and although some of the infants' mothers I spoke to were older than this, many had started having children some time ago (thereby skewing the results somewhat). In terms of parity, just over half of the women (13) had one child, a third (9) had two and the remainder (3) had three. Only five women in this sample were no longer breastfeeding at all; they were generally the eldest and had the eldest children.[4] The children being breastfed ranged from newborn to 4½ years old (again, many women I interviewed were breastfeeding older children). The oldest breastfeeding mother was 47 (her child was 4), and the youngest was 23 (her child was 14 months).

Three quarters of women in the sample (19) were married, whilst three were cohabiting. Only two were single (because they were divorced). In response to whether they were working at the time of being questioned, only one answered yes. Four said they were on maternity leave; eight said they were working part-time; and twelve said they were not working outside the home at all (11 of the 25 gave their profession as 'Mum'). Five of women had postgraduate qualifications, two thirds held a degree, and the remainder had either A levels or GCSEs.

Only fourteen of the women were born in the UK, although the vast majority of their children were born there. The women came from a wide range of places: Malaysia, Finland, France, Australia, Germany and Ireland as well as the UK, though these findings are not put to explicit use here. Women's comments about raising a child in the UK are perhaps more poignant when prefaced with comments about perceived differences (and, of course, when they problematise a homogeneous idea about being 'British'). Twenty-two listed themselves as white; one woman classed herself as Chinese, another Hispanic, and one Irish. All women spoke fluent English and answered questions in English.

In sum, the mothers at LLL meetings in London were in the vast majority white, in their thirties (on average, 35), well educated (to university level or equivalent) and married (see Appendix 2 for a summary of these results). There was little discernable difference in these demographics between the attachment mothers and the general LLL group, save that the attachment mothers were less likely to be working outside the home than those in the main sample. In addition, the average age of children being breastfed in my general sample in London was 18 months, whereas average age of children being breastfed in the attachment sample (excluding children under 1 year old) was 2¼ years. There was no gendered correlation with extended feeding – that is, there was no notable difference in the numbers of boys or girls being breastfed in this way.

Reflexivity

The dual approach of participant-observation within groups and more intimate one-to-one interviews meant that gaps emerged between these two methodological approaches – descriptions of full-term breastfeeding as enjoyable and empowering, fleshed out by accounts of the experience as tiring and difficult (the two are of course not mutually exclusive, and their overlap is indicative of an intensive mothering framework). For example, Amelia wrote the following about her experience of breastfeeding:

> *Questionnaire*: What has your experience of breastfeeding been like, both at the beginning and over your child's life?
>
> *Amelia [33, breastfeeding her almost-3-year-old son]*: At the very beginning it was painful (bleeding nipples due to latch attempts that struggled due to C-section & epidural) and exhausting (three to four hours each morning spent nursing, in addition of course to breastfeeding throughout the day and night), and it was extremely powerful in creating a strong bond and asserting my place as primary caregiver amid the clamouring of relatives for 'involvement.' Over time it has developed from what I saw as a means of nutrition into an essential parenting tool, reducing in frequency dramatically (down to about ten times per 24 hour period by the age of 1 year and now about five times per 24 hour period) but increasing in importance in handling parenting challenges, used for soothing hurts, handling transitions, reconnecting after a noisy period, or trouble between us, etc.

This (written) narrative – although frank about difficulties – has a glossy feel to it (note the importance of breastfeeding with 'handling transitions'). This woman also struggled over a period of months to come to terms with the fact that her son was going through a phase of hitting and biting other children. As she put it, in tears at one meeting and apologising to the collected group, 'I feel so embarrassed. I thought that if I breastfed him he would turn out to be a nice gentle boy, and here he is acting like a thug.' To use Goffman's terms, Amelia's different accounts, shared through this dual methodology, function as elements of her 'impression management' (Goffman 1959). As a form of embodied accountability then, these accounts are deeply political:

> Giving an account is a political act because it either confirms or un-settles whatever happens to be taken for granted as the world of nor-mal appearances. To be 'accountable' for one's activities is both to explicate the reasons for them and to supply the normative grounds whereby they may be 'justified'.... The intersection of interpretive schemes and norms does not occur in the abstract. *Instead, this intersec-tion is enacted by embodied beings whose sense of identity is rather confirmed or denied through processes of accountability.* (Willmott 1996: 28; empha-sis added)

Non-participant Observation

At virtually every meeting, I was asked whether I had been breast-fed as a child, whether I would breastfeed my own children, and for how long (and for almost everyone I tell about my research, this seems to be the first question). I was happy to share the fact that I had been breastfed by my mother, though I worried in due course that this would bias women towards me in an unintentional way. Certainly, in what seems an odd claim, I am glad to have written a book about breastfeeding without having ever breastfed a child; nor indeed given birth to one. Not being a mother afforded me a 'research space' that allowed me to learn about infant feeding from a less involved position (perhaps in many ways akin to other an-thropologists who approach their fieldwork as 'cultural novices'). I was allowed to ask the obvious questions without being perceived as sharing a moral consensus about the importance of breastfeeding for the maternal experience. I could even ask about how it felt to breastfeed, in the most basic and physiological terms; what a blocked duct was; how many times a day a baby would need feeding; why milk does not dry up after a week when a mother is only feeding occasionally; whether it was true that milk could squirt out of your breasts at the sound of a baby crying (it can, apparently). For many of the women with whom I worked, the importance of breastfeed-ing is a product of the culture of intensive motherhood, which binds breastfeeding to notions of optimal care and maternal diligence. My own position as an outsider to this culture meant that I was not au-tomatically one of 'us' (breastfeeder) or 'them' (formula feeder). I problematise this non-participant observation further in Chapter 8, which looks at feeling.

Accounts

Why Breastfeeding?

During the course of research, I – perhaps as a woman without children – was often surprised by the somewhat dogmatic assertions about the merits of breastfeeding and the lengths to which women would go to in 'achieving' it (echoing the work of Schmeid et al.). I met several women who, unable to breastfeed at the breast directly for various reasons (such as surgery), used lactation aids that enabled them to feed their baby with their (expressed) breast milk through a tube at the nipple; others recounted stories of bleeding nipples, immense pain and lots of distress in the early stages of breastfeeding. I was interested, then, in why breastfeeding was so important to these mothers.

In the questionnaire conducted with my informants, the three most cited reasons for feeding one's child with breast milk were that it was 'best', that it provided immunity from illness, and that it was 'most natural'. This response from Alice – a 47-year-old mother to 25- and 15-year-old sons and a 5-year-old daughter, whom she had just weaned – was typical (if somewhat more extensive than others):

Questionnaire: Why was it important to feed your child with breast milk?

Alice: It was the food made especially for my baby.
Breastfeeding brought us closer together and helped us get to know one another.
It taught my child to trust me and feel safe.
I only wanted the best for my child.
I couldn't give my baby a substitute knowing I was withholding the best.
I believe it is a child's birthright.
I wanted to give my child the best food available.
I wanted them to have healthy immune systems, good dental formation, and general good health.
I wanted my children to be mentally and socially healthy.
I wanted to be able to feed my child whenever he needed to be fed. I could not bear the thought of him being distressed waiting.
I am aware of the dangers of artificial feeding.
I want my children to have healthy attitudes to food for life. This involves them being active rather than passive feeders from birth.

Note that she mentions 'wanting to give her children the best' several times, and that she is very well versed in the arguments frequently heard at LLL meetings and in breastfeeding advocacy literature.

As to why it was important to feed their children at the breast, women most frequently mentioned a desire for optimal bonding or closeness with their children. Half the women mentioned 'love', whilst a third spoke of experiencing a sense of confidence that their breasts were serving their 'true purpose'. Alice continues:

> *Questionnaire*: Was it important for you to feed your child at the breast?
>
> *Alice*: Yes. It is what nature intended and any other way of feeding is a very different experience for a child. I don't know what adverse effects there could be for a child not breastfed, and was not going to take the responsibility of denying them the experience.

For Anastasia, breastfeeding crystallised her mothering:

> *Questionnaire*: How would you describe breastfeeding your child?
>
> *Anastasia [38, mother of 5- and 2-year-old daughters, breastfeeding 20-month-old daughter]*: The ultimate expression of motherhood.

'Still' Breastfeeding?

Whilst women's decision to breastfeed their children is certainly an interesting subject for research, this study focused on women's reasons for *continuing* to breastfeed beyond 'normal' timeframes (i.e., beyond a year). This framing, perhaps, reveals my own prejudices. When I asked my informants why they were 'still' breastfeeding, attachment mothers would usually answer by turning my question around: why would you stop? Breast milk and the immunity and nutrition it provides continue to be beneficial at whatever age it is consumed, they told me:

> *Charlotte*: The mums who decide to feed for a long period of time.... What would be the arguments for that?
>
> *Jane [25, Leader applicant, breastfeeding her 16-month-old son]*: It's just as nutritious as the day they were born, so that is great. And just things like, last week I was really ill, and I couldn't get out of bed, and we just stayed in bed and breastfeeding, and he was still getting all the nutrition he needed, and that would probably apply if he was a bit older too ... and when he is upset or anything, or poorly, it is just such a comfort ... Mmm. Yeah, there are lots of health benefits there for the mother as well, and for the child.

There was also a definite sense that women felt that by mothering in this way, they were building 'secure emotional foundations' for their children:

> *Sally* [*42, breastfeeding her 1-year-old daughter*]: … I hate to sound preachy. But we really hope that by the time she is a teenager, she will have had her fill of being held and touched and breastfed, and be quite a secure person.

Being able to comfort a toddler having a tantrum, or a hurt child was said to be the most gratifying reason for continuing to breast-feed, one that made the work of mothering considerably easier.[5]

Given breastfeeding was such an important part of their relationship, women also frequently mentioned as an advantage the fact that children could talk about it. They hoped that since these children were slightly older, they would also be able to remember this happy time:

> *Charlotte*: So, you said that when you were pregnant you would feed probably for six months…?
>
> *Judy* [*39, breastfeeding her 4- and 2-year-old daughters*]: My mother breastfed for nine months, and my reference was that really, she said 'once you were big enough to start undoing my buttons I knew it was time to stop'. And so every month I did after that, with [my child] really, as I had more time to think about it, I thought it's a bit sad my mother didn't experience this. Because an older child communicates about it, talks more about it, it's likely she will remember it … we spend so many hours doing it, and there is so much conversation around it.

So children enjoy breastfeeding, and mothers also find it relaxing:

> *Charlotte*: So why are you breastfeeding?
>
> *Signe* [*30, Leader applicant, breastfeeding her 3-year-old son*]: I guess I continue to do it because it is important for [my son] and, and because he asks for it … it obviously makes him feel better, he talks about it a lot, and says a lot of really sweet things about it. And because I find it an easy way to comfort him and to calm him down, and if he is feeling bad about something and doesn't always know how to talk about it, we can just take the time to sit down … and it's totally different to a year ago … I guess, I enjoy it [too], I enjoy the chance to sit down and in the evenings [whilst breastfeeding] I can sit down and read a book or something.

Finally, continued breastfeeding made women feel that their bodies were capable and productive, expressing their femininity in a very powerful way. One mother of a 14-month-old son, still predominantly breastfed, spoke of her pride at growing and nurturing him 'all by myself'. 'This is what I was designed to do,' she said.

Experiences

In the questionnaire, Patricia (30, breastfeeding her 1-year-old son) summarised the best and worst things about long-term breast-feeding:

Best

1) The feeling of giving and receiving love when breastfeeding. The closeness and comfort you can give, especially at the beginning when communication is so limited. [He] cried a lot after he was born for the first few months, and the quiet times of feeding him and being able to make him happy was a lifesaver for me emotionally.

2) Being able to comfort [him] when he is really upset

3) Seeing him grow and thrive on breastmilk

Worst

1) Being bitten. He started to bite me when teething was really bad for him and now he does it as a bit of a habit. I find it really difficult and am trying to find ways of stopping him.

2) Being totally responsible for getting him to sleep

3) Back ache from hours spent lying on my side feeding him at night

I asked other mothers whether there were any disadvantages to breastfeeding their older children:

Lauren [42, breastfeeding her 30-month-old daughter]: Waking up at night! I can't even remember how many times she wakes me up and she nuzzles into me.

Victoria [38, breastfeeding her 5- and 3-year-old sons and her 18-month-old daughter, and at this point pregnant]: Like I say it's just so painful with her [Victoria is trying to reduce the amount of breastfeeding her daughter does as she is now pregnant again, which can make the nipples more sensitive]. So I am trying to put her off. I'm trying to find other ways of distracting her, you know, when she wants it, finding other things for her, and I only feed her when she is really desperate. Because ... she will feed and not want to stop, even when it looks like she is fast asleep, so I say ... stop stop, and I can't even get my finger in to stop it, as she will bite me ... you probably know, when you are pregnant you just sort of have this thing where you get to your limit and you don't want anyone to touch you at all. And you just say 'that's it, I just want you off' [but then] the more she doesn't want to go off, probably because I am making her feel like that the more ... she is feeling like holding on, and I am thinking 'go away'.

One interesting thing Sally commented on was the lack of 'intimacy time' she got with her husband:

Sally [*42, breastfeeding her 1-year-old daughter*]: There is another thing about co-sleeping and breastfeeding that we find very difficult. She won't be put down on her own. I need to lie down with her. She needs nursing to sleep, and wakes up if I get up. So I have to stay there. Which means that we get very little private intimacy time.

Some more minor problems were connected with extended feeding – one had to watch what one ate and drank and couldn't necessarily dress as one wanted (since few speciality breastfeeding clothes exist, except in maternity sizes). These were generally seen as minor sacrifices:

Mette [*35, breastfeeding her 3-year-old daughter*]: It just seemed right, it just came naturally when I got pregnant, that I didn't want to drink [alcohol] … I just felt sick. It's not like I found it difficult. But then even when it stopped, I drank a few glasses in my pregnancy, so that just came naturally. When she was quite tiny, I wouldn't drink. [Now] maybe two in the evening, as I am going to sleep with her, you know. It just feels right not to do it, not a big thing to discuss. Overall, I wouldn't swap it for anything.

Case Study

Fleshing out these narratives is an extended account from one of my informants – Lauren, a married, white, 42-year-old woman, originally from Belgium, breastfeeding her 2½-year-old daughter, her only child.[6]

I 'woke' up in the morning at around 5 – not bad, as it's often earlier. It's actually been three years now since I've woken up naturally; [she] always seems to be wriggling around well before I would otherwise wake up! She had a quick breastfeed and a cuddle and I managed to persuade her to stay in bed for another hour and a half or so.

But it's impossible to keep her in once it gets properly light outside – so we got up and I went and made some tea. I tried not to wake my husband who was on the sofa, but he had to get up for work anyway, so he got up and had a shower and I made tea for us all. I'm drinking jasmine tea at the moment. It's not quite the same kick as caffeine, but it is refreshing in this hot weather! I made breakfast for [her] once her father had gone – we had some really good wholemeal toast and butter, which she ate very happily. She likes food she can pick up and help herself to, rather than having it shoved down her throat. I've always had an interest in nutrition, and I think it's best to give children proper food – so, we have butter not margarine and brown bread not white, for example.

After eating I pottered around the house with her, tidying things up from last night, folding up the sofa bed, and putting the sheets in the wash. We shared a bath, I got her dressed and she played around as I got ready. No sexy underwear, lipstick or jewelery any more, because she tugs at my earrings, and can't feed so well with normal bras. And if I wear lipstick it goes all over her.... But it still takes me a while! We went to the LLL meeting, which was at half past ten on the other side of town. I think she got a bit flustered about having to put her shoes and coat on, so we had another quick bit of 'booby' before we left, which made our leaving a bit late.

We walked slowly to the tube – I carried her in her sling for the last bit as we were going to miss the start. She wanted to walk, so she was a bit annoyed, but she got distracted by the escalators, which she thinks are good fun. Luckily she didn't ask me to feed her on the tube, which she has done in the past. It's not that I mind, it's just that you have days where you can't be bothered with all the stares.

The meeting was great – nice to see everyone again. We were talking about 'common problems with breastfeeding' which is a bit unnecessary for me now, but it's still nice to meet new mums and hear the new research. There's one mum who has just moved near our house actually. I find I really miss it if I don't go every month ... you recharge your batteries until the next time. Of course, [she] wanted feeding whilst we were there. Normally she wouldn't want any in the middle of the day, but when she sees all the other babies doing it then she is reminded about it. She only had a little bit. I think she probably wanted a cuddle more than anything else. She also had some of my lunch after the meeting – hummus and carrots, some bread, cheese and some home made fruit cake that Sian had brought.

I carried her all the way home in her sling because she was pretty worn out after running around with the other children. We stopped off in Waitrose on the way home though and she sat in the trolley for that. She knows all of the assistants there, and they all know her. She 'helps' me with the shopping – I let her pick out some of the fruit we are going to have in the house, and she likes talking and pointing to the man at the deli counter. They've got some really nice nuts and seeds in there too, so I picked up some of them for me.

I actually had a bit of a migraine developing, but managed to get home before it got too bad. I usually just lie down in the dark for a bit and it fades away. I realised I had forgotten to hang the sheets out before we left, so I did that then closed the curtains and crashed out! [She] was very good – she came and lay with me and I think we both slept for a little bit on the sofa.

In the afternoon, when I felt a bit better, I let her watch her CBeebies video whilst I got up and started thinking about supper (I know I shouldn't have, but sometimes it's just easier!!) I decided to make pasta with pancetta and Savoy cabbage – the best use for Savoy cabbage after using the leaves as compresses for engorged breasts! I actually decided to make the pasta myself, as I love proper cooking. It took quite a while, and [she] wanted to help quite a lot, but she likes using the machine, so we had a bit of fun doing that. But rather annoyingly, it turns out that she doesn't like pasta after all, so for all my hard work to try and feed her good stuff, she ended up with baked beans! Not ideal, but she was so hungry by that point I couldn't argue. They are Waitrose organic!

We went and sat outside in the garden when she'd finished supper – I got the washing in, and we played a bit in the sand pit with her toys. She likes burying things and then 'finding' them at the moment.

I checked my emails while she watched a bit more telly (I know! but I don't get anything done otherwise), and then I tried to put her to bed at around 8. She wouldn't lie down without me, of course, so I lay there for a bit trying to get her to settle. She was sort of falling asleep on me, but trapping me underneath her at the same time! Every time I tried to move away she realised of course.

In the end, I heard my husband come in at about 9 after his meeting, and I got up to see him. She woke up and started hollering, so she came and joined us in the sitting room. Things are a bit tricky at the moment with our sleeping arrangements. We all start off in the big bed and then seem to shift about so as to maximise sleep! He is on the sofa a lot of the time, but neither of us mind – we see it as a small sacrifice for a few years. It does cut down on your intimacy time as a couple, but it just means you have to be more inventive!

Anyway, he ate some of the pasta and then watched some TV. We chatted for a little while, but [she] started being grizzly so I went to bed with her. She went off to sleep fine this time – and so did I. I still wasn't feeling that good. She only woke me up a few times in the night – once for a feed, though I told her she could only have the bottle of water, as I'm trying to stop night time feeds entirely, as we might try for another baby.

Contextualising Full-Term Breastfeeding

This account, which focuses on the day-to-day realities of full-term breastfeeding, is far removed from the way the practice is generally portrayed by public outlets. Whenever I explain my research – to peers, colleagues or friends – the usual response is some sort of surprise, if not disgust. ('Breastfeeding a 5-year-old? That's gross!') The majority of people I speak to do not know that a woman can lactate for such an extended period of time, let alone that so many of them would want to. There is generally a sense that there is something strange – possibly even perverted – in women's 'need to be needed'.

(See also Dowling [2009a, 2009b] on the stigmatisation women experience when breastfeeding for extended periods of time.) To convey a sense of this, I put 'full-term' breastfeeding into the context of the contemporary UK by citing a typically sensationalist *Daily Mail* article on the subject, published in June 2008:

> **Her friends are horrified, but the woman who still suckles her five-year-old insists: I'll breastfeed till they're EIGHT!**
> Stella Onions doesn't worry about people staring.
>
> Whether sitting outside a cafe or walking round the park, whenever she breastfeeds her two children, she ignores the women gawping and men brazenly pointing her out to their friends.
>
> Even in her own home – the only place she now lets her son and daughter feed from her – she barely cared when one friend turned away, unable to watch as they suckled.
>
> But such reactions are hardly surprising; the babes sucking at this middle-aged mother's breasts are toddlers aged five and three years old.
>
> For many, breastfeeding at this age is unnatural, crossing the boundaries of normal maternal behaviour. (*Daily Mail,* 13 June 2008)

The picture published with the story was captioned: *Mother knows best: Stella Onions breastfeeds daughter Josephine, aged five, who says she does not want to stop until she's married, and four-year-old Zac* [sic].

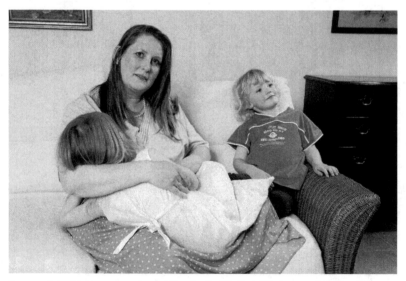

FIGURE 3.1. Picture accompanying *Daily Mail* article, reproduced with permission, Alistair Heap / Solo Syndication

In a similar vein, the comments below come from a BBC Radio 1 Internet forum following the screening of the Channel 4 documentary *Extraordinary Breastfeeding* in 2006, which featured one mother (Veronika Robinson, editor of *The Mother Magazine*, a natural parenting magazine, LLL member and prominent figure in the attachment parenting community) breastfeeding her 7-year-old daughter. Radio 1, the BBC's 'new music' station, has a young target audience.[7]

[Emphasis added] **Women who keep going until their kids are nine years old [sic] feature in Channel 4's documentary Extraordinary Breastfeeding … Does that thought freak you out? Or are we too uptight?**

Leila: I think breastfeeding beyond 1–2 yrs is a bit bizarre and *becomes more about the mother's psychological want, not a child's biological need*. Women continue to lactate because of the stimulation through feeding, not because of a nutritional need of their offspring. And there are many other things children learn to take comfort in as they grow up and learn independence from their parents – to justify the continuance of breastfeeding as a source of comfort sounds like a mother that can't let their baby grow up and doesn't want to let their child go.

Jody: I started puberty early and at the age of 9 was noticing the opposite sex … I had not before considered breastfeeding a child of that age, *surely it is going to develop some strange ideas about life?* In this day and age we are seeing pregnancies at 13, only 4 years older. We don't know what the moral implications are but I imagine they will have an effect later in life. What is next, what is going on with society and when do people know when to draw the line?

Gaz: This is sick! How exactly do these mothers think they are helping their children's development? You wouldn't let your 10-year-old walk round with a bottle with a teat on it would you? *Here's an idea – get all their friends and their parents round to show them what they do – let's see how normal they feel then.*

Jenny: This is just wrong, ok fair enough babies need nutrients and the goodness that comes from a mother's milk when they are born but past 6 months they are perfectly capable of producing the nutrients through other means and *this is just abuse to a certain extent.* Who in their right mind would think that it is 'right' and 'necessary' for a 3-year-old or worse 8- or 9-year-old drinking from their breast?! It's absolutely disgusting.

In a more sober fashion, one mother I spoke to – who had gone along to an LLL meeting but decided it wasn't for her – sums up many of these concerns:

Charlotte: Why isn't it for you [breastfeeding to full term]?

Sarah [*breastfed both daughters for a year*]: I also have a few issues about, well, I just question sometimes is the mother doing it for them and their emotional need, or are they doing it for the child's needs? And I think, I don't think the child needs it nutritionally, you know it provides a very strong bond, but then I think it can become a sort of a crutch ... but also, also sorry, sorry this is sort of challenging all my prejudices and stuff, but I have sort of read about it in the case of the single mother and her only boy child, you know, which I always feel a little strange about, and I think in some ways the boy child has replaced a partner, I mean, I don't sort of think that every woman that is breastfeeding is sitting there thinking sexual thoughts, because it just isn't like that, I don't think that is at all what happens, and I just think, I wonder if it is emotionally beneficial to the child.

Breastfeeding, Body Boundaries and Individuality

My informants, who were well aware that many viewed them as 'sick' or even 'abusive', regarded full-term breastfeeding and attachment parenting in contemporary Britain as hard because 'separation is endemic to our society' (Sally). In an interview, Veronika Robinson told me, when I asked why it was that people might have a problem with the sight (or idea) of a child breastfeeding beyond infancy, that 'to have a baby attached to the mother through breastfeeding is just the opposite of what our society is encouraging'. This is not confined to older children, then, but is an anxiety that intensifies over time if the child is not considered to be 'separating' from its mother:

Veronika: It's a cultural thing. If you look at our society everything is designed to separate mother from child; it happens, you get pregnant and you have a scan, and that is the first thing, that separation, it is telling the mother not to trust her own intuition, you know a mother has to rely on something outside to tell her about herself. And then the baby is born and the cord is cut straight away ... everything right from those beginning stages, 'get the mother away from the baby'. It's everything; the sleeping, the walking – we celebrate milestones of separation. So if you have a baby that is attached to the mother through breastfeeding, that is just the opposite of what our society is encouraging.

Leticia added that mothers who do not 'separate properly' from their children are considered suspect. I asked her whether there was a pressure on women to stop breastfeeding after a certain age, and she replied:

Leticia [36, 3½-year-old son, breastfeeding her 2-year-old daughter, emphasis added]: I think socially there is a pressure to 'get out and get your life back'. I think there is a pressure there, to get the baby in its own room at a certain point, to get it out of the bed at a certain point. To create a certain distance between you and the baby, *I think that is thought of as very healthy and if you are not doing that you are considered to be depriving your child, or not quite adjusted somehow.*

For Marilyn Strathern, the individuality of persons is the first fact of English kinship (1992b: 14). She writes, 'It is when persons become visible as individuals that the English feel they "relate" to one another' (1992b: 49). To follow her argument, one might say that to 'relate' to each another, separation of the mother from the child (as part of this process of individuation) must be cultivated so that 'attachment' can begin. This separation is catalysed through techniques of visualisation typical of foetal scans (Petchesky 1987), as much as in the moment of birth.

Indeed, this is not a transition confined to a moment; rather, it is processual. In her essay 'Parts and Wholes', Strathern notes that people do not arrive as individuals but are made so through processes of socialisation (and, arguably, separation), which in turn enables their participation in social life (a plurality of individuals):

The English person conceptualised as an individual was in one important sense incomplete. ... There always appeared to be 'more than' the person in social life. When the singular person was taken as a unit, relationships involved others as like units. Social life was thus conceptualised as the person's participation in a plurality. As a result, an individual person was only ever part of some more encompassing aggregate and thereby less than the whole. Where a prototypical Melanesian might have conceptualised the dissolution of the cognatic person as making incomplete an entity already completed by the actions of others, our prototypical English took the person – powerfully symbolised in the child that must be socialised – as requiring completion by society. (Strathern 1992a: 86–87)[8]

Thus most mothers in my sample perceived the problem with long-term breastfeeding 'in society' as people's understanding of it as (bodily) evidence of the child not really being separate from the mother – a relic from the time when a baby is unable to act autonomously and as such precluding, one could argue, either the mother or the child from participating in the plurality of society as individuals.

The link between the body with definable boundaries and self-hood is long established in Western philosophy. These bodies, which are the property of the subjects who inhabit (or 'are') them, maintain a distinction from other bodies by managing the transgression of their boundaries (such as in the flow of substance between them). Breastfeeding is therefore a challenge to the notion of the individual body, since the ejection of milk from the breast does not sit easily with the 'fortress' metaphor of the body/self (Martin 1998).

Martin has written about women's inability to be an 'individual' (one who cannot be divided) as a deeply political fact. Quoting Franklin and Haraway, she says:

> pregnancy is precisely about one body becoming two, two bodies becoming one, the exact antithesis of individuality (Franklin 1991: 203). Donna Haraway (1991: 253n) explains: 'Why have women had so much trouble counting as individuals in modern western discourses? Their personal, bounded individuality is compromised by their bodies' troubling talent for making other bodies, whose individuality can take precedence over their own.' (Martin 1998: 134–135)

In pregnancy, a woman's body/self becomes doubled – and breastfeeding, particularly for 'extended' periods, serves as a reminder of this ability to reproduce and transgress these boundaries. Martin continues:

> not only the state of motherhood but also women's state of health in general, their failure in many ways to achieve the male norm of the self as a defended castle, leads to the same effect. Whether leaking fluids through ducts and membranes (which simultaneously allows penetration of the foreign into the body) or permitting the body to turn against itself, this porous, hybrid, leaky, disorderly female self is the antithesis of the sharp-edged man. (Martin 1998: 135)

Defence Strategies

Perhaps not surprisingly then, 'judgement' was the challenge women most commonly cited in regard to their full-term breastfeeding:

Charlotte: We were talking at the group about the documentary [that featured Veronika Robinson]…

Sandra [*Leader, 35, breastfeeding her 4-year-old daughter*]: I did see it, yes. My in-laws were a bit like 'that's disgusting', especially with the older children. They are still a bit uncomfy about the fact I still do it. 'Don't do it in front of us, and we won't comment' sort of thing. It has been quite good in terms of generating discussion; you know, a way for us to broach it and explain why we're doing this.

Many women have simply lied to people, or at least kept their breastfeeding as discreet as possible. As Katy put it, 'I do tell people if they ask me directly, but to be honest, I find it easier to avoid the topic.' This included health professionals. Others used jokes to divert the attention – referring to *Little Britain's* 'bitty' sketch, (a comedy show featuring character who breastfeeds as an aristocratic adult) or suggesting their children would still be breastfeeding when they went to university. Some women talked about being 'strong-minded' and the criticisms being 'like water off a duck's back':

> *Lauren [42, breastfeeding her 2½-year-old daughter]:* I really couldn't care less, I am a strong-minded woman and I couldn't care less. Nobody has ever told me anything. And I have actually never had anyone come up and say anything to me. I mean, I get some little remarks from distant family or something, about 'oh my god, you're still breastfeeding?' but I joined LLL which has been a wonderful support because they really dispel myths and they really inform, and its not perfect, nothing is perfect, but I have got so much information.

The analysis now turns to La Leche League, exploring how it operates as a network offering women support for their full-term breastfeeding, and a social identity formed around a shared set of mothering values.

Notes

1. In the London case, 40 per cent of mothers fed their infants formula. A hospital report lists the ethnic groups of its approximately 5,500 mothers per year as: white – 50.1 per cent; black – 37.7 per cent; Asian – 7.6 per cent; other – remainder. The (private) Parisian hospital did not have these figures available.
2. Central London (plus a newly formed Stoke Newington branch of the Central London group); East London, Havering, Woodford, South East London, Bexley and Bromley, Croydon, South West London, and Haringey and Barnet. I visited those groups easily accessible by London (TfL) transport. There are now two new groups: LLL West London and LLL Clapham. In Paris there were eight groups, including the anglophone group, Bievre, Bambins des Colllines, Hauts de Menil Montant, 'Madellleine,' Paris Sud, Paris Seine and Paris Ville. There are now two more

groups: Paris Nord and Vaugirard, neither of which was established at the time of research.

3. Some women I *interviewed* were younger or older than the ranges given here, and were breastfeeding older children. I restrict my demographic profile to those who filled out questionnaires, as they provided more comprehensive data.

4. Having weaned their children, these women continued to come to meetings to share their experiences with younger mothers.

5. One woman told a vivid story of comforting her toddler when he ran into a plate glass window – the only thing that could help him with the pain was breastfeeding, which also stemmed the bleeding. The image she described – blood pouring from his mouth down her shirt – was particularly memorable.

6. I asked Lauren to talk me through a typical day in our interview; I have edited out my responses here. Lauren also added some details by email later.

7. http://www.bbc.co.uk/radio1/news/newsbeat/060201_extraordinary breastfeeding.shtml Retrieved 20 December 2006. The page has since expired.

8. I do not enter into a discussion here about the oversimplification of a Euro-American, bounded self and an othered 'relational' one. See Carsten's *Cultures of Relatedness* (2000: 83) for a good summary.

Chapter 4

LA LECHE LEAGUE
PHILOSOPHY AND COMMUNITY

A Typical Meeting

I'm in a suburb of London, lost and late. I consult my map. After getting my bearings and walking from the bus stop for what seems like hours, I finally arrive at my destination: a semi-detached house with a small garden at the front.

I ring the bell, thirty-five minutes after the scheduled meeting time. A woman comes to the door. 'Charlotte?' 'Hello,' I say, 'you must be Janet?' She ushers me in, waving away my apologies for being so late. 'The first thing you have to realise,' she says, 'is that there is no such thing as being late for a La Leche League meeting. Don't worry at all – we're just making tea for people anyway; so you haven't missed anything'. Until this point, Janet, an LLL leader, and I have only communicated by email. She let me know that I would be very welcome to come along to her group's series meetings – provided I introduce myself as a researcher and am aware that the meeting is a space for women to discuss their breastfeeding concerns. 'Just let people talk to you,' she says, 'I'm sure they will.'

Janet shows me into the sitting room of the house, where a group of mothers and children are assembled. I notice a huge spread of food in the adjacent dining room – homemade cakes, bread, celery sticks, fruit, and later on, cheese and hummus. I add my own offering – dried apricots – to the selection as I take off my coat and retrieve my notebook and Dictaphone from my bag. A little table in another corner holds a few books for sale, as well as the group library and a collection tin for donations. On the wall is a small, rather elderly handwritten poster that says: 'Attend to your own family's needs; Keep side conversations to a minimum; Keep confidences; Take only what you want from this meeting!'

I turn into the sitting room, where three women are waiting with their children. All of them are white and between about 25 and 45 years old. I introduce myself by saying that I am a student writing a thesis about breastfeeding. (I ask to record parts of the meeting, and take notes throughout. What follows here is a 'hybrid' account from notes taken during several meetings in the same group. See Piper and Sikes (2010) for a discussion of this methodology in the protection of anonymity.) 'That's great!' says one mother: 'We can talk about breastfeeding as much as you want!' Janet comes through from the kitchen followed by Alice, who lives here and is the hostess for the meeting. They bring a tray of tea – both herbal and caffeinated. We settle into a vague circle – some on chairs, others on the floor, whilst the children play in the middle with the toys.

Janet suggests we get started. It's 11.15 a.m. – 45 minutes after the scheduled time. 'Welcome to the North West London La Leche League group.' (The names of the group and participants have been changed.) 'I know most of you know this already, but I'm going to do this properly for the new people.' She nods towards me and the mother holding a very small baby. 'So, hello! I'm Janet, the group leader, and this is Alice, to whom we are very grateful for hosting.' Janet continues: 'La Leche League (or, the 'milk' league) is an organisation which was set up in the States by a group of women who wanted to help women breastfeed their babies. It is based on the idea of mother-to-mother support, by providing support for breastfeeding women. We do this by giving mothers information about breastfeeding (not advice!) so that they can decide what works best for their families. We believe that mothers are the experts on their own babies, but that sometimes we could all do with reassurance about what we are doing.' Janet pauses to dust off a child who has fallen over, cooing at him as she does so. 'The group will be 50 years old this year, and is generally recognised as the foremost authority on breastfeeding in the world. We work as an NGO with the UN and WHO and we have active groups in over 60 countries. But this doesn't all happen out of thin air! We depend on our members for support, so if you are interested in joining, please talk to Megan, who is our group treasurer and librarian. Apart from the warm glow you'll get from signing up, you'll also receive discounts on our books, be able to borrow from our library, which is in the corner there, and get a regular newsletter from LLLGB.

'Before we introduce ourselves, there are a few announcements. The toilet is upstairs, where you are welcome to change your babies if you need to – please look after their needs first. What else? Oh yes, the area conference, which is happening next month: I will be driving from here, so let me know if you would like to have a lift. And finally, it is National Breastfeeding Awareness week, so there are some events with which the group will be involved, at which we could do with some volunteers. It would be really good to have some real-live breastfeeding mothers to come and take part in "The Big Feed" in the park next Saturday.'

She looks at her notebook. 'The subject for this week's meeting, which is the fourth and final one of the series, is "Nutrition and Weaning", and we are here to iron out any concerns you have.' (It is worth reiterating at this point that 'weaning' is a somewhat ambiguous term used to refer to ceasing breastfeeding entirely, as well as continuing to breastfeed alongside the introduction of other foods.) 'Please remember – I know, I say it every time – that at this meeting we will discuss a variety of ideas. Some of them might be new to you, even a bit surprising. Remember that you are free to take what you like and to leave what you don't. There is no one way to care for your children – only you know what works for you and your family. Now, why don't we go around the circle and introduce ourselves and our children by saying something about what we hope to get out of being here?'

We are six adults and four children in total. We start with Alice. Alice says that she has three children, all breastfed. Two of them are now grown up, though her daughter, Katy, who is 5, has only recently been weaned. Katy plays and shares her toys with the other children as the meeting goes on. Alice has been active in the group for the last twenty years and enjoys hosting meetings and sharing experiences with new mothers. The next mother, Amy, is here for the first time with her 4-week-old baby, June. She says she doesn't really want to know about weaning quite yet, but is here because she is having terrible trouble with mastitis, which makes breastfeeding very painful. She has spoken to Janet on the telephone but is here to get some more practical help. Janet promises to take her upstairs for a 'one to one' on positioning once the discussion has drawn to a close. Ruth, who is 24, is next: she is here with her 1-year-old son Edward, whom she describes as 'a greedy little man, still mainly breastfeeding at a year old!' I introduce myself, and my project, passing round a few copies of the information sheet for my study. Next is Megan, age 41, who is here with Christopher, her 4-year-old son, and wants to talk about 'W-E-A-N-I-N-G him' (in this case, cease breastfeeding). She doesn't want Christopher to hear her say 'weaning', as he has learnt to associate the sound with being refused 'nummies' (the word he uses when he wants to breastfeed).

Janet thanks us all and apologises for not introducing herself properly. She has three children, all breastfed: Mark is 14, Mary 11 and Jo 6. Janet discovered LLL only when Mary was born, so Mark was breastfed for only three months – 'because of all the support I wasn't given,' she says, to knowing laughs in the rest of the group. (Although she doesn't mention it in the meeting, I find out later that Janet's youngest child, Jo, who is on a play date today, still breastfeeds from time to time, usually just before going to bed).

Janet kicks off the discussion by reading aloud a few sections from *The Breastfeeding Answer Book*, LLL's guide for breastfeeding mothers. She comments that in our society, it is unusual to see a child breast-feeding beyond 6 months old, but that in other societies around the world this is the norm. The World Health Organization, she says, puts the average global age of weaning at 4 years old and recommends breastfeeding in developed countries in conjunction with other foods for up to two years or beyond. I jot this down, surprised that this is a recommendation for developed countries. She comments that 'there is a social expectation that women will want to get their babies on the bottle by 6 months', but that LLL exists, in part, to help women who want to continue breastfeeding past 'normal' (she makes quotation marks in the air) lengths of time.

As she speaks, Megan is being nudged by Christopher, who is say-ing he wants 'nummies'. She sighs at him, but slips up her t-shirt as he pulls down her bra and attaches himself to her nipple. She gives him a quick smile. He stands up, holding on to her breast with both hands as she continues to listen to Janet. Amy, here for the first time, looks at me and then looks away.

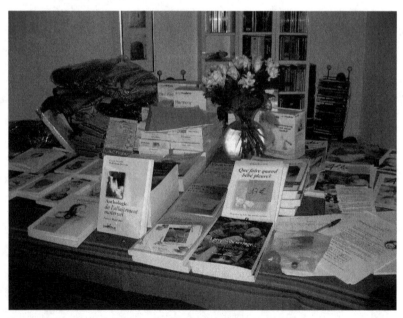

FIGURE 4.1. A group library, Paris, 2006, author's photo

I notice that Edward, Ruth's son, is wearing a T-shirt that reads: 'Care Instructions: Hand Wash Only; Love Unconditionally; Breastfeed as Required'. Ruth laughs about it when she sees me reading the words: 'I know, it was the least militant one I could find on the Lactivist site – some of them are even worse! But I really like them – and I do find it helps with the comments.' She takes the opportunity to pick up the conversation. 'It's funny really. Before I came to LLL, I believed everything the doctor told me about feeding him.' She pauses because other people are loudly agreeing. 'He said that by 6 months, breast milk stopped being nutritionally valuable, and that I ought to put Edward on a formula with sufficient iron content. It's so ridiculous! These people have a duty to educate and support women, not spin out twaddle like that. I didn't listen to him, but it did upset me that someone with such power was so ignorant. I actually told him the next time I saw him how wrong he was about the iron, because the iron in formula milk isn't actually bio-available to the baby anyway.' Again, Amy catches my eye and looks a bit bemused. Ruth is currently training to become an LLL Leader, and throughout the meeting comes out with more facts about the relative merits of breastfeeding over formula feeding. Janet effectively closes the topic, saying that 'Many mothers have found that breastfeeding beyond 6 months has been nutritionally adequate for their children, in conjunction with other foods, so it's probably worth discussing this with your doctor the next time you see him.'

In time, the conversation turns towards Megan's problem. Because she wants to have another baby, she needs to cut down on feeding Christopher so that her periods will return and she will be able to conceive again. Being 41 years old, 'time is sadly of the essence'. (She says a lot of this in a code language so that Christopher doesn't understand her words.) The problem, she says, is that she wants him to lead the weaning himself, because she wants the process to be as natural and un-traumatic for Christopher as possible. 'He seems to really need it still', she says 'but is it ok for me to say no sometimes, or does that mean it's not child-led?'

Before Janet can answer, someone else starts talking. 'I remember having exactly the same problem,' says Alice. We listen to her tale of this situation eighteen years ago. 'It is absolutely not wrong to put your needs on a par with your child's,' she says: 'They are not little princes! You need to make breastfeeding work for you, as well as for them. Child-led does not mean you can't negotiate.'

The conversation continues on this theme for a while longer – another hour, in fact – before Janet suggests that we call the meeting to a close and have some lunch. 'Thank you all for coming, and please help yourselves to what's on the table.' She takes Amy upstairs to make sure she has got her baby latching on to the breast correctly.

Over lunch, I speak with each of the women more informally. After
the close of the meeting, I notice that the conversation broadens to
topics outside of breastfeeding. We talk about local schools, which
Megan is eschewing in favour of home schooling Christopher. Ruth
talks with Megan about a local cranial osteopath that she recommended, thanking her for the suggestion; others discuss a nice local
park that has just opened up. Alice tells me about how the group has
changed over the course of her time with it: 'We get all sorts of people
now. Not like the old days! I remember seeing a woman that came
with nail varnish for the first time and all of us being shocked – how
does she have time to put on nail varnish, we were thinking.'

La Leche League's Philosophy

La Leche League's philosophy was crystallised early in its history, to
allow dissemination of the organisation's values:[1]

- Mothering through breastfeeding is the most natural and effective way of understanding and satisfying the needs of the baby.
- Mother and baby need to be together early and often to estab-
  lish a satisfying relationship and an adequate milk supply.
- In the early years the baby has an intense need to be with his
  mother which is as basic as his need for food.
- Breast milk is the superior infant food.
- For the healthy, full-term baby, breast milk is the only food
  necessary until the baby shows signs of needing solids, about
  the middle of the first year after birth.
- Ideally the breastfeeding relationship will continue until the
  baby outgrows the need.
- Alert and active participation by the mother in childbirth is a
  help in getting breastfeeding off to a good start.
- Breastfeeding is enhanced and the nursing couple sustained by
  the loving support, help, and companionship of the baby's father. A father's unique relationship with his baby is an important element in the child's development from early infancy.
- Good nutrition means eating a well-balanced and varied diet of
  foods in as close to their natural state as possible.
- From infancy on, children need loving guidance which reflects
  acceptance of their capabilities and sensitivity to their feelings.

This chapter addresses the values behind this philosophy, exploring some of its contradictions. Gorham and Andrews (1990) make a

useful division, which is followed here, focusing on four philosophical aspects in turn. They argue that La Leche League can be said to have:

> 1) Support for 'complete' breastfeeding; 2) Support for constant and continuous mothering and for a style of baby and childcare which follows the lead of the child rather than the caretaking adults; 3) Support for the family as the most significant unit in society; 4) Support for 'natural' as opposed to technological methods of childbirth [and child rearing]. (Gorham and Andrews 1990: 243–244)

Complete Breastfeeding

That the child should determine both the frequency and duration of breastfeeding continues to set LLL apart from other breastfeeding support groups. At the time the league was founded, it was far more common that a mother be encouraged to schedule feeds, most typically with formula milk, as part of optimal 'scientific motherhood' (Apple 1987, see Chapter 2). The use of formula milk is discouraged, as is – though to a lesser degree – the use of bottles of expressed milk, unless absolutely necessary, as these are considered to interfere with a child's desire to nurse at the breast.[2] Solid food is ideally introduced once the child shows an interest (such as a willingness to pick up foods, chew, etc.) at some point during the first year. To this end, 'baby-led weaning' has recently become a topic of interest in the parenting world (see Head 2011; Rapley 2006).

The LLL philosophy not only advocates exclusive reliance on breast milk in the early months of the child's life but also supports 'full-term' breastfeeding, generally well into toddlerhood (or beyond), saying that ideally the breastfeeding relationship will continue 'until the child outgrows the need'. Gorham and Andrews quote the first edition of *The Womanly Art of Breastfeeding* to answer the question of when a baby should stop breastfeeding: 'Let the baby do it. Let him nurse until he wants to stop' (Gorham and Andrews 1990: 245). Only more recently, since the 1980s, has the league explicitly offered information and support for women who want to breastfeed their toddlers, for which it has become known amongst other support groups.[3]

Mothering

The third point in LLL's philosophy states that a baby has 'an intense need to be with his mother which is as basic as his need for food'. Gorham and Andrews argue that LLL understands mothering as a vocation, backed up by psychoanalytic theories that oppose mother-infant separation. Indicative of the social value with which mothering is imbued, Marian Thompson, one of the founders of LLL, is quoted in *The Womanly Art of Breastfeeding* as saying, 'the kind of people we produce is crucial to the direction our world takes. Raising a loving, caring child is the most important contribution any of us can make to the progress of the world' (LLL1: 2004: 14).

It was common during meetings to hear women say that they had been encouraged (by doctors, generally) to schedule their child's eating patterns for fear of 'spoiling' the baby and 'making a rod for one's own back'. LLL strongly disagrees with this suggestion, arguing instead that responding to a child's needs is the most effective way to create independence. Similarly, it is believed that a child should not be disciplined in harsh or authoritarian ways; rather, he or she should receive 'loving guidance' from parents. The child's feelings and capabilities should be respected, and mothers are discouraged from pushing their children to develop too quickly. The 'intense need' to be with the mother is not thought to cease after the early months, but to continue well into childhood. The league considers itself the 'child's advocate', which sits well within a broader framework of intensive motherhood, validating women's identity work through child-centred forms of care.

The Family

One interviewee answered the question of 'what LLL is all about' by saying: 'It's about families, really. It's about family togetherness.' Indeed, as Gorham and Andrew note, the idea that the nuclear family is the building block of society is a central tenet of LLL philosophy. In terms of breastfeeding, a father is considered most useful when he acts a supporter of the mother-infant 'dyad'. In many ways LLL can be seen as upholding very traditional male/female roles taking place in domestic/public spheres accordingly. On the other hand, LLL has always encouraged fathers to be involved in childcare – such as by bathing their children or soothing them by holding them and singing to them. At the time LLL was founded – 1958 – this was considered radical.

As noted, he founders of the league were acquainted through the Christian Family Movement, a Catholic organisation encouraging family values, and there remains some cross-pollination of values today (Ward 2000). For example, LLL implicitly encourages large families – many examples in its publications depict such families, and it is frequently remarked that the seven founders had fifty-three children between them (with one woman having eleven). During the course of fieldwork, two women mentioned their Christian faith as an important part of their parenting philosophy. This religious background is not stressed in the literature, for fear of excluding mothers who would otherwise seek support for breastfeeding. Thus, although there is an underlying pro-life, traditional family message, the league is careful not to 'ally itself with any other cause' than breastfeeding.[4]

LLL advocates family activities that involve all members, rather than those that exclude children. Many women talked about how they would take their children with them when they went out for dinner, or would prefer simply to have a 'date night' at home with their partners. One of the most notable areas of family togetherness is the advocacy of the 'family bed', whereby all members of the family sleep together until children are ready to sleep alone. This is advocated on the basis of not only making breastfeeding easier in the early days (saving the mother the difficulty of having to get up for night-time feeding and enabling her to respond as quickly as possible to her child's cues) but also strengthening relationships with fathers, who otherwise have little contact with their children due to being at work or similar contingencies. The league's *Purpose and Philosophy* states:

> LLL believes that breastfeeding, with its many important physical and psychological advantages, is best for baby and mother and is the ideal way to initiate good parent-child relationships. The loving help and support of the father enables the mother to focus on mothering so that together the parents develop close relationships which strengthen the family and thus the whole fabric of society. (LLLI 1998)

Nature

A final thread running throughout the LLL ethos is a celebration of nature. Although one high-ranking member of LLL told me that they tried to avoid talking about the 'naturality' of breastfeeding, as it is a problematic term, 'natural' is found in almost all LLL texts. Breastfeeding, states the philosophy, is the most 'natural and effective' way of feeding babies. 'Natural' childbirth, eschewing interventions in the process of labour, is implicitly advocated to encourage optimal breastfeeding ('active participation by the mother in childbirth is a help in getting breastfeeding off to a good start'). Home birth has long been advocated amongst many LLL members, though, again, this is never done explicitly.

As Gorham and Andrews (1990) observe, much of this philosophy comes through the work of Grantly Dick-Read, a London-based medical doctor and social reformer who favoured non-medicated childbirth and prophylactic approaches to pain relief. (It was on the basis of his work that the Natural Childbirth Trust (National Childbirth Trust, since 1961) was founded in 1956 by Prunella Briance [Kitzinger 1990].) LLL also advocates 'natural' family planning, stressing the benefits of the 'natural' spacing that occurs when breastfeeding continues at a sustained level (a further point of congruence with Catholicism). Furthermore, foods that are in 'as close to their natural state as possible' are considered ideal. In recent years, this philosophical belief has intersected with wider cultural trends towards ecologism – 'natural' food, 'green' solutions to modern life, and so forth. Moscucci (2003) notes that 'natural' childbirth and parenting as a philosophy has long served as a political and cultural critique aimed at the various crises of modern society – be they industrialisation, capitalism, materialism or urbanisation. The solution to these problems is seen to lie in a return to nature, variously understood as the rural, the primitive, the spiritual or the instinctive (Moscucci 2003; also see Chapters 6–8).

The Founding of LLL Great Britain (LLLGB)

LLLGB started as an LLLI 'area' in approximately 1971. The first leader in Britain was an American woman based in London. The first British LLL group, however, was set up by another American leader in Leicester. It was held at the home of a local mother who became one of the first UK-accredited leaders.[5]

Being an LLL area meant being an administrative division of La Leche League International – and hence subjecting all top-level decisions to ratification by leaders in the United States (even, in the early stages, the accreditation of a new leader). Over the following ten years, as the group expanded, UK members voted to become an LLL 'affiliate'. When this happened in 1984, the UK branch of the organisation gained greater autonomy. This process was not without ruptures – in the interim period between formation as an 'area' in the early 1970s and final accreditation as an affiliate in the 1980s, a group of mothers broke off from LLL group to set up the Association of Breastfeeding Mothers (whose founder was the original American LLL leader in the UK).

LLL is managed by volunteers at every level and is regulated through the Charities Commission. At the time of research, LLLGB had around 170 accredited leaders, 75 local groups, and 150 LLLGB-led peer counsellor programmes throughout Great Britain. As noted, there were approximately 900 paid-up members of LLLGB, though many more (nearly 8,000) attend the meetings (LLLI 2008). LLLGB offers a UK phone line, staffed by leaders. It publishes a bimonthly magazine for members, *Breastfeeding Matters*. LLLGB members also receive the LLLI publication *New Beginnings*. Leaders receive the magazine *Leaven*, and LLLI also profiles the latest research on breastfeeding in *Breastfeeding Abstracts*, a publication for professionals that members can also sign up for.

Paradoxes of Appeal

How, and why, did La Leche League take off in the UK during the 1970s, nearly two decades after its inception in the US?

A Feminist Organisation?

The prevailing strand of feminism in the 1970s was arguably one of cultural feminism. To quote Stewart, this is the idea that 'there are fundamental, biological differences between men and women, and that women should celebrate these differences.... Cultural feminists are usually non-political, instead focusing on individual change and influencing or transforming society through this individual change. They usually advocate separate female counter-cultures as a way to change society but not completely disconnect' (Stewart 2003, in Aegnst and Layne 2010: 71). To this end, the LLL's *Purpose and Philosophy* states:

> LLL further believes that mothering through breastfeeding deepens a mother's understanding and acceptance of the responsibilities and rewards of her special role in the family. As a woman grows in mothering she grows as a human being, and every other role she may fill in her lifetime is enriched by the insights and humanity she brings to it from her experiences as a mother. (LLLI 1998)

As Weiner notes, La Leche League's ideas about mothering, developed in the 1950s, make it an interesting organisation in the context of second-wave feminism and women's entry into the labour force in the latter half of the twentieth century: 'La Leche League reconstructed mothering in a way that was both liberating and constricting and so ironically offered both prologue and counterpoint to the emerging movement for women's liberation' (Weiner 1994: 383). The representations of mothering in *The Womanly Art of Breastfeed-*

ing promote a traditional heterosexual parenting set-up, at the same time recognising mothers as the experts on their babies and encouraging self-empowerment and enhanced autonomy in the face of (so-called male) authorities such as doctors (noted by Hausman 2003: 158). LLL also offers support to women who wish to be stay-at-home mothers, which is perceived to be in short supply in wider society. Mothers and babies are encouraged to be together regularly and often, especially in the early months, and women are told that mothering (rather than employment or domestic chores) should be their priority.

In the leaders' handbooks, the prerequisites for leadership state that a woman should manage separations from her baby 'with sensitivity', though what this really entails is much debated. Only in 1981 did LLL first make any mention of working mothers in *The Womanly Art of Breastfeeding*. Today, whilst there remains an implicit message that work is best avoided, LLL is aware of the need to help working women breastfeed their babies and accordingly offers information on expressing breast milk. This remains a divisive topic, and many leaders I met felt that this information compromised the league's philosophy of mother-child proximity.

The appeal to traditional gender roles, legitimated through the needs of the infant, is deeply problematic for many feminists. Yet LLL understands breastfeeding as providing an expression of women's 'natural power' (echoing the claims of natural birth advocates). As Penny Van Esterick puts it, breastfeeding 'confirms a woman's power to control her own body and challenges medical hegemony' (Van Esterick 1989: 70). As a 'womanly art,' breastfeeding is understood by LLL to be a means by which women can reclaim their bodies, boost their sense of self-esteem and resist conventional authority in all its forms (Lee and Bristow 2009).

LLL therefore rejects portrayals of women's bodies as primarily objects of male consumption (Bobel 2001: 135). Asserting the role of breasts as nutritive, they understand themselves to be pioneering feminists. Bodies are a source of empowerment, something to be 'enjoyed'. As this mother commented:

Sandra [Leader, 35, breastfeeding her 4-year-old daughter]: No one has a problem with breasts to sell newspapers.... But society has this thing about not using them for their intended function. And the way our society is into undermining women's confidence in their own bodies.... What we can do is amazing. I don't have a body that our society celebrates, but I have managed to grow a child and nurture her for four years, and that is amazing. I have always struggled with my weight, but stop telling me my body isn't adequate, because it can do this amazing thing.

These tensions are obviously inherent to a maternalist philosophy, which reflects broader tensions between feminists – contradictions that have remain unresolved: 'Exalting women's capacity to mother has contradictory implications for efforts to end women's subordination, as some use a woman-centred perspective to empower women whilst others use biological essentialism to constrain women's opportunities' (Blum and Vandewater 1993: 297). Bobel sums up this tension when she refers to LLL's philosophy as advocating a 'bounded liberation' (2001: 131).

Unlike other authors who pursue this form of enquiry, Hausman (2003) is interested in how considering breastfeeding as a practice of embodied motherhood could change feminist approaches to maternity, as well as to philosophical considerations of sexual difference, and this is a lens I have found productive here: 'Both the espousal of traditional mothering *and* feminists' excoriation of LLL as a conservative organization mired in 1950s domesticity emerge from a social context that does not recognise women as having a biological relation to their offspring that is different from men's (that is, physiological rather than genetic)' (2003: 158). In considering La Leche League's attention to breastfeeding within maternal domesticity, she complicates the arguments of feminists who claim that LLL's adherence to traditional and domestic maternity is congruent with a gendered, capitalist order (i.e., ensuring that male employees remain ideal workers by having family structures to support them). She suggests that, rather than simply toeing the traditional line, LLL contributes to contemporary debates about women's roles as mothers and workers.

At the same time, Hausman takes a particular position in the debates around breastfeeding, saying that she became frustrated, as a breastfeeding advocate, with 'the feminist collusion with the idea that in order not to induce guilt in mothers who don't or can't breastfeed, we shouldn't argue for its benefits, or even acknowledge that breastfeeding has a biological benefit at all' (Hausman 2003: 6). Other feminists, such as Joan Wolf (2011), question this very certainty, which associates formula feeding with a large range of health problems. As discussed in Chapter 2, she argues that in many areas (for example obesity, IQ and psychological development) the evidence is varied and highly inconclusive. What each position agrees upon is, once presented with a sober assessment of the pros and cons, the need for more material support for women who *do* choose to breastfeed in practical, rather than verbal terms. To this extent, they both also recognise the gendered subject positions women occupy in debates around public health, often being held individually responsible for wider structural inequalities.

Science

Education and support for mothers are key concepts for LLL and fit well with its feminist orientation. The use of science is held to increase women's authority – a belief reflected in the growing amount of clinical evidence in LLL publications. Other scholars have drawn attention to the contradiction of breastfeeding advocates' co-option of the language of science – an ironic move, because their usual discourse is that of *anti*-rationality, medicalisation or expertise. In her study of La Leche League, Ward (2000) describes how LLL was established as a movement prioritising the expertise of mothers over that of the medical profession, and the 'natural' qualities of breast milk over the scientific claims made by formula manufacturers. Here we should be careful to note a distinction between medicalisation and scientisation (Hausman 2003). The group can crudely be said to be 'anti-medicalisation' but 'pro-science'. As Hausman puts it: 'With their strong ties to medical advocates and advisors, the League could not resist all the facets of scientific motherhood, yet their palpable ambivalence about the doctor's role in making decisions is clear' (Hausman 2003: 169).

Indeed, this ambivalence is more than evident. LLL's *Purpose and Philosophy* states:

> La Leche League was founded to give information and encouragement, mainly through personal help, to all mothers who want to breast-feed their babies. While complementing the care of the physician and other health care professionals, it recognizes the unique importance of one mother helping another to perceive the needs of her child and to learn the best means of fulfilling those needs. (LLLI 1998)

Whilst promoting mother-to-mother support, LLL is clear that it is not a replacement for health care professionals, though it does urge women to be upfront about the care they wish to receive and offers them support in doing this – 'a doctor should be there to help not direct', says one leaflet advising pregnant mothers. This is not a simple distillation of the intensive mothering injunction; rather, it is a challenge to the notion of professionalised parenting. If anything, LLL encourages women to question expertise:

Sunanda [31, breastfeeding her 2-month-old son]: One time I was in the clinic with this South American woman who was breastfeeding her 22-month-old child and the Health Visitor made a point of saying 'what are you doing that for?' in front of everyone, so this woman took him off. And I would have said, 'do you mind? It is none of your business!' And I was appalled really, I mean, I'm going to breastfeed him [her son] as long as he wants it, no matter what any health professional says.

Yet the league, always conscious of the potential for appearing as 'quacks' (as one leader put it in our interview), has therefore made conciliatory efforts towards the medical profession without losing sight of its own values. LLL formed a medical advisory board for editorial approval of materials and advice on specific problems, and physicians were invited to speak at conferences. Indeed, the very founding of the group was in conjunction with medical doctors, as husbands of two of the founders were medics sympathetic towards breastfeeding. The group has also run a 'physicians' seminar' every year since the 1960s (although this appeared to be in jeopardy at the 2007 International Conference). Accordingly, and in congruence with the increasing research about the benefits of breastfeeding, there has been growing acceptance of the league in the professional and medical community, to the extent that the tenth step of UNICEF's Baby Friendly Hospital Initiative encourages women to use lay support groups such as LLL.

It is useful to look at LLL through the lens of professionalisation, and the way voluntary groups have increasingly gained political capital on such a basis. The league recognised that health professionals and leaders, particularly those with medical training, were showing growing interest in professionalising their breastfeeding skills. Indeed, there is a career to be made out of breastfeeding support today. As a result, early in 1982, the LLLI Board mandated the establishment of a lactation consultant program, now known as the International Board of Certified Lactation Consultants (IBCLC). LLL writes:

The primary purpose of International Board Certification is to benefit the public by setting standards for the lactation consultant profession. Board Certification provides a credential for lactation consultants that validates their expertise, knowledge, and skills. Employers, colleagues, and consumers can be assured that the designation 'IBCLC' identifies a member of the health care team who can provide substantive breastfeeding care and services as well as skilled technical management for breastfeeding problems. (LLLI 2000: 52–53)

LLL and Attachment Parenting

A significant proportion of the values LLL promotes are compatible with those of 'attachment parenting', and amongst breastfeeding groups LLL is known to be welcoming and supportive of women who practise this style of care. In the late 1980s, William and Martha Sears coined the term attachment parenting (AP) in *The Baby Book*. They argue that AP is

> an approach to raising children rather than a strict set of rules. Certain practices are common to AP parents; they tend to breastfeed, hold their babies in their arms a lot, and practice positive discipline, but these are just tools for attachment, not criteria for being certified as an attachment parent.... Above all, attachment parenting means opening your mind and heart to the individual needs of your baby and letting your knowledge of your child be your guide to making on-the-spot decisions about what works best for both of you. In a nutshell, AP is learning to read the cues of your baby and responding appropriately to those cues. (Sears and Sears 2001: 2)

The Searses argue that the optimum way of caring for a baby keeps the mother and child in extended physical contact ('attached'). Drawing on historical arguments, they say that this is really just 'common-sense' parenting: 'This style is a way of caring that brings out the best in parents and their babies. Attachment parenting has been around as long as there have been mothers and babies. It is, in fact, only recently that this style of parenting has needed a name at all, for it is basically common sense parenting we all would do if left to our own healthy resources' (Sears and Sears 1993: 2). The 'tools' of attachment parenting given by the Searses are given in Table 4.1:

TABLE 4.1. The ABCs of Attachment Parenting
The Tools of AP, Sears and Sears 2001: 4

When you practice the Baby Bs of AP, your child has a greater chance of growing up with the qualities of the As and Cs:

As	Bs	Cs
Accomplished	Birth bonding	Caring
Adaptable	Breastfeeding	Communicative
Adept	Babywearing	Compassionate
Admirable	Bedding close to baby	Confident
Affectionate	Belief in baby's cry	Connected
Anchored	Balance and boundaries	Cuddly
Assured	Beware of baby trainers	Curious

The 'B's' enable parents to tune in to their baby's 'cues', which in turn enables them to parent appropriately.

Today, Attachment Parenting International (API), a not for-profit organisation founded in 1994 by LLL members in the US (Lisa Parker and Barbara Nicholson), is a global movement that exists to support parents who practise AP. Drawing heavily on the work of the Searses, their website states: 'API provides parents with research-based information, tools and support that affirms positive, healthy parenting, and helps parents create the kind of legacy that they can be proud to bequeath to their children: family strength, reduced conflict, feelings of love and being loved, trust and confidence. A legacy of love.' (API 2009) The API's eight principles read:

> Prepare for Pregnancy, Birth, and Parenting
> Feed with Love and Respect
> Respond with Sensitivity
> Use Nurturing Touch
> Ensure Safe Sleep, Physically and Emotionally
> Provide Consistent and Loving Care
> Practice Positive Discipline
> Strive for Balance in Your Personal and Family Life

Many women in LLL were familiar with the work of the Searses – indeed, they were among the most frequently mentioned authors during research. But it would be wrong to say that LLL simply provides the breastfeeding expertise whilst the Searses (or API) offer the more general approach to parenting. Full-term breastfeeders within LLL may hold more conservative or Christian values, not necessarily congruent with the values of attachment parenting, or simply breastfeed for long periods because they find it easiest for their families (the relationship between values and practices, as stated at the outset, is not straightforward, and not all long-term breastfeeders are attachment parents). Nevertheless, there is clearly considerable overlap between the two groups' philosophies – given that API was founded by LLL leaders and close working relationships exists between LLLI and the Searses – who, now branded AskDoctorSears.com, appeared as honoured guests at the recent fiftieth-anniversary LLLI conference.

LLL for All Mothers?

One criticism of LLL has been that it addresses only one type of mother, and certainly, my data seem to reflect these clichés. Several mothers I interviewed commented on this fact:

Charlotte: What sort of demographic was it at the meeting you went to?

Sarah [38, breastfed both daughters for a year; went to one LLL meeting and never returned]: Exactly what I expected! You know, middle class white, slightly on the hippy side of things. I mean, sorry ladies! I guess I am a middle class white too, but, yeah, I would have been really quite surprised to see an Asian woman, or a Bangladeshi woman for example. About 30, 40, my sort of age… older mum end.

LLL is considered to be apolitical and unconcerned with mothers in lower socio-economic strata, an opinion that was prevalent amongst health professionals and mothers outside of the league. Typical of the academic criticism on this subject, Blum writes: 'Although La Leche League is an organization dedicated to maternal nurturance, it demonstrates a lack of political action for low income mothers and enhanced medical, welfare and anti-workfare policies needed by increasing numbers of women' (Blum 1999: 91–92). Yet LLL's focus has always been on providing support for women who have *already chosen* to breastfeed. LLL has not, for example, taken a specific stance towards government policy on, say, maternity leave (although it operates on a quasi-official level in coalitions such as the Breastfeeding Manifesto Coalition). This has led to it being seen as caring only about those who have the resources to stay at home or manage their workplace to accommodate breastfeeding or pumping.

There is a tension here, in that LLL has fairly fixed views about what the ideal mothering relationship looks like – making it hard to offer 'support' to women who do not endorse this vision:

Charlotte: Do they appeal to certain strata in society?

Jane [Leader applicant, 25, breastfeeding her 16-month-old son]: Yeah.

Charlotte: Should they change that?

Jane: No, because it would be a different organisation. I mean, they would have to have a completely different sort of philosophy [one that wasn't about mothers and babies being together often]. I mean, sometimes I think it doesn't reach everybody… they do help everybody, but it is a certain type of person at the meetings. Certain people are drawn.

In an interview, I discussed LLL policy with the Chair of Council:

Charlotte: Should you be making efforts to appeal to all members of society?

Jemima [Chair of Council]: See the word you used there? I think we should be 'accessible', not to 'appeal to'. Rather than making ourselves into something for other people ... we should be making our-selves available to all mothers. You know, there is no mother we would turn away, that our communication channels are wide and varied so that any kind of mother can access us. ... Having said that, we have recognised that there is a whole section that isn't going to reach us in the way that we are at the moment. Which is why we have the peer-counselling programme. That is a much clearer way of reaching the less advantaged. It is clear that our groups do not meet all elements of all sections of society ... I am very proud of the peer counselling programme.

The peer counsellor programme (PCP), piloted in the Nottingham area during the 1990s, trains individuals to train others to become breastfeeding counsellors. LLL-accredited leaders train health professionals in breastfeeding support skills, which they then pass on to women who want to become 'peer supporters' in their local area. Trainees draw on a set of materials, including the *Breastfeeding Answer Book* and *The Womanly Art of Breastfeeding,* as well as a curriculum and other assessment materials, though they do not receive LLL leader accreditation. The website explains: 'Health professionals are trained by LLLGB's PCP Team to become administrators of this highly successful programme. They are then enabled to recruit, train and support mothers to become breastfeeding peer counsellors in their local areas' (LLLGB 2008).

Once the peer counsellors have been trained,

> [they] help change attitudes to breastfeeding in their areas, empowering themselves and those around them. Mothers empowered by the peer counselling course often to move on to employment or study. They become, for example, play workers, health care assistants, midwives ... and some decide to train as La Leche League Leaders. They know though, that their greatest achievement is having improved the lives of their children, through breastfeeding. (LLLGB 2008)

Evaluation of the scheme showed that women were twice as likely to breastfeed in areas with an LLLGB PCP than in comparable areas without such a programme. Despite LLL's having fewer than a thousand dues-paying members, its influence is now felt far and wide, since the vast majority of breastfeeding counsellors in the UK are and will be trained with some form of La Leche League material. Use of LLL materials on a national scale represents a considerable advance for the group.

We have seen, then, that as a global organisation, La Leche League has been the foremost provider of information, education and support for breastfeeding to women for over the last fifty years. Yet the league is guided by a very specific philosophy that poses some interesting questions around feminism and empowerment, which are taken up in later chapters. The next chapter explores in more depth how LLL creates and sustains a sense of community, particularly for women practising the attachment parenting philosophy.

Notes

1. From LLLI publication No. 300-17, 'La Leche League Purpose and Philosophy'.
2. 'Cross-nursing' of more than one baby by one woman is not encouraged officially (on the grounds of health risk and interruption of the unique bonding process) but is a practice I saw occasionally amongst group members (often sisters).
3. Gorham and Andrews cite one of the first information sheets on extended nursing, published in 1982 by S. Diamond: 'Still Nursing?' LLLI Information Sheet, no. 97 (August 1982).
4. So whilst several founders wanted to take a stance against abortion in the early days of the league, this was not ratified (Interview with founder, LLLI Conference, 2007). On its purpose, LLL states: 'The League's purpose is distinct. This singleness of purpose does not prevent interaction with other organizations with compatible purposes, but La Leche League will carefully guard against allying itself with another cause, however worthwhile that cause may be' (*La Leche League Purpose and Philosophy*, LLLI Publication No. 300-17).
5. Information from interview with long-standing leader.

Chapter 5

'Finding My Tribe'

For Douglas, '[n]ot just any busload or haphazard crowd of people deserves the name of society: there has to be some thinking and feeling alike among members' (Douglas 1986: 4). What is needed, she argues, is a shared symbolic universe – a social basis of cognition. This chapter outlines the ways in which the attachment mothers I worked with came to be involved with La Leche League and explores the processes by which social groups are formulated and maintained through shared values and practices. The argument is that 'norms' within the group can have a coercive effect with respect to behaviour, an important aspect in the creation of community.

Why Do People Come to La Leche League Meetings?

In the London groups, just over a quarter of the women who filled out the questionnaire responded that they had come to LLL to fix a physiological problem such as breast pain, sore nipples or poor infant weight gain. In general, these women were not at LLL because they had (originally) a specific interest in the philosophy of mothering through breastfeeding, full-term breastfeeding or attachment parenting. Rather, they had selected LLL from a range of resources listed in leaflets or books distributed to mothers by agencies concerned with infant feeding.

Indeed, many breastfeeding support groups are available to women, though no other has a philosophy quite as explicit as LLL's. Other groups do not promote breastfeeding as a central element of the mothering experience or a source of identity work to such an extent. One NCT breastfeeding counsellor made the following observation:

> *Jo*: I'm a member of a lot of organisations, but La Leche was seen as very radical, no question.
>
> *Charlotte*: Back then [the 1980s]?
>
> *Jo*: Oh yes, and even now to some extent … I mean, it's funny; the big breastfeeding mums I meet [through NCT] would find more in common with La Leche meetings than NCT where women often go back to work, where they would pump and where they would maybe mix feed by a few months and let babies sleep all night. Whereas La Leche was about the sling and attachment parenting and that sort of thing.… And they were seen very much as very radical … their aim was about breastfeeding. But now it has changed, because LLL got involved in peer support. I went to this thing a few weeks ago and they are involved in all these projects you know, in Hackney, Lambeth and stuff and it's great! I mean, it's not under the La Leche name, but it means the ideas are becoming mainstream again. All the better.

For women who have come to LLL by chance, it operates as a solution finder to breastfeeding problems. In general, women would come to a few meetings, ceasing once their problem had been resolved. One leader wrote about this in an email:

> I would just like to add that when I started going to LLL meetings in … 1998, there were a lot more new mothers with new born / under 6 months present than there are now. At each meeting, there was always at least one mother who had not been before. The turnover of mothers attending meetings was much greater with mothers attending just one meeting. However, there was a hard core of mothers who regularly attended. Numbers were generally around the 20 mark on average. Now, meetings tend to comprise solely of the hard core group, with an occasional new mother. I think this is because of the increase in breastfeeding drop-ins [organised by other groups]. (Personal communication, LLL Leader, 14 May 2006)

It is the 'hard core' or 'attachment mothers', who often came to the group when their babies were 6 months to a year old, that are of interest here. A quarter of the mothers in the UK sample came after six months of breastfeeding an infant, as did many of the mothers I interviewed (generally, women met over the course of several monthly meetings). They wrote that they came 'to find other people continuing with breastfeeding when others were stopping' (5 women) or to 'find like minded people' (15 women). When asked to explain a bit further, women mentioned needing 'support' for continuing to breastfeed beyond normal lengths of time, and a desire to find people to socialise with, as mothering was sometimes a lonely business. Amelia even talked about how interactions in her NCT group made her feel 'suicidal':

> *Amelia [33, breastfeeding her almost-3-year-old son, emphasis added]*: So I was quite involved in an NCT antenatal group, especially when he was small ... and I just realised that they were going down a different path, I realised that they were having a very different experience to me, and I found that very depressing actually. Because they would talk about breastfeeding as a prison sentence. And I didn't realise why I would feel upset when I left ... we were doing the same thing, but they were having different experiences. They were doing the whole Gina Ford routine thing, they weren't taking any confidence in themselves ... I can say this now looking back on it, but at the time *I just felt suicidal every Thursday* ... about a week later, I phoned LLL, and one of the counsellors that you met actually ... yes, she was like, come along.... Well *it was just like coming home to my own people or something.* And after that, well, I've just sort of come to each meeting that I can. Because it just presented me with *a different picture of ... what it meant to be a mother* where I could accommodate my child without feeling like I was 'giving in' to something. A common phrase that comes up is that 'you are making a rod for your own back' so that is how I got involved in LLL.

The support LLL offers to women in situations like this cannot be underestimated. Women would talk of how 'La Leche League saved my life, as I know it'. Often, after months of escalating exclusion and accountability ('having to fight my corner'), women described LLL as a haven where they didn't constantly have to explain themselves:

> *Sandra [Leader, 35, breastfeeding her 4-year-old daughter, my emphasis]*: And they were pretty much all bottle-feeding [at the mother and baby group]. And I think they were mostly there just to talk to each other, whilst the babies sat there in push chairs with the dummies in their mouths. I don't remember seeing anyone else, interacting with their babies unless they were crying. I thought *this felt really alien to me. It felt uncomfortable.* Getting to LLL was great ... I didn't have people telling me how to 'get my life back'. This *is* my life, you never get back to how it was before – it never goes back to what it is before you have a child.

Clearly, many women felt isolated in relation to other mothers, having decided to breastfeed beyond 6 months of age:

> *Sally [42, breastfeeding her 1-year-old daughter, emphasis added]*: Well, I'd done NCT and the few mummies in my group had all stopped, or were stopping breastfeeding ... I think there were two of us, and the other one was about to start weaning. *So I felt quite alone ... and it was more than that, it wasn't just the breastfeeding; it was the whole attitude toward child-rearing as well.*

It was not only the fact that women had decided to carry on with breastfeeding, then, that made them feel different from the mothers around them – it was their 'whole attitude towards childrearing'.

'Finding my tribe'

Arguably, people are drawn to organisations like LLL when they feel marginalised by dominant social practices. These groups gain adherents because a positive sense of identity can be developed where perceptions are shared: interaction both aids an individual in finding explanation for a life event (breastfeeding), and helps forge a collective identity through the development of a particular discourse and a set of perceptions and ideas (Allsop, Jones and Baggott 2004). Indeed, many women I spoke with talked of how they had made lifelong friends through LLL, particularly if they were long-serving leaders. For many women, La Leche League's philosophy (demonstrated at group meetings) was like 'coming home'. Sally says that she 'felt like she had met her 'tribe':

> *Sally [42, breastfeeding her 1-year-old daughter, emphasis added]*: I just felt a bit isolated ... they are wonderful my [NCT] group.... But soon I just wasn't part of it ... but there was a conversation I just wasn't part of. *I just felt like the extreme freak in the corner.* And also *it's lifestyle, the whole attitude* ... some of them were doing the controlled crying thing, it all goes together and I just find that so alien – I just wanted to meet other mummies who were doing what I was doing.... *I feel like I have met my tribe – even though we are very different people, I am normal there. I am not an extremist.*

It was interesting to consider the extent to which LLL gave women the chance to express parenting styles that just 'felt right' to them, and to what extent women had, by coming to LLL, opened their eyes to a way of parenting they hitherto had not known existed. Perhaps not surprisingly, they tended to mention a combination of the two:

Charlotte: So did you have these ideas already, and you found women with similar views, or did going encourage you to think about new things?

Mette [*35, breastfeeding her 3-year-old daughter*]: A bit of both ... but probably a bit more of the latter. I knew I should breastfeed ... and I knew I wanted to do that for at least a year ... so I think I picked up a lot, that it is normal and it is acceptable to breastfeed for a year. ... And just knowing that you can go to the meetings and that it is ok, and be reminded, you know, you are normal, when you have lots of people asking you.

The meetings were, then, a space where women were allowed to be normal and at the same time somewhere to learn what was normal. Some women narrated this as a revealed truth, known all along 'in my heart' but articulated, or 'allowed', by the LLL philosophy:

Charlotte: Was coming to LLL like finding 'your sort of people', or was it a bit of a surprise, some of the things you saw there?

Pippa [*Long-serving leader, emphasis added*]: Probably a bit of both ... suddenly knowing that it was ok to want to be with your baby. Society tends to say that you mustn't let a baby change anything, and to have somebody say, of course you want to be with your baby, that was ... *something I felt in my heart all along, but couldn't actually articulate it.* And the pressure from other people to go away and leave my baby was very great. *So it was sort of like coming home.* This thing about the mother and baby relationship made sense to me, in a way that nothing really had before ... that was how it felt at the time. And still feels. I probably was thinking about these things before I came across them, but not in a very conscious way.

LLL was a great source of support for women who felt ostracised for breastfeeding older children, particularly when it put their own 'extremism' into perspective:

Charlotte: Is it nice to be with other mums doing the same sorts of things?

Amelia [*33, breastfeeding her almost-3-year-old son*]: Yes, [to be with] like minded people ... it is a big spectrum ... there was me thinking that I was being ridiculous for feeding him at 15 months, and here is someone feeding a 7-year-old. ... It puts things in perspective.

So being 'normal' is a relative term here. Within an LLL meeting, breastfeeding beyond a year is certainly 'more' normal than amongst the wider population. Seeing the more extreme ends of the spectrum puts women's individual practices into a broad continuum and offers them a framework within which to rationalise their own choices.

There are, of course, several types of normal. One may be statistically normal, but idealistically anomalous (e.g., divorced in a culture that values a marriage as the ideal household unit but where the majority of marriages end in divorce). As Tiefer (2004) says, the 'need to be normal' is a question of social conformity: 'The average person uses the word in a kind of cultural-statistical way. How people feel about themselves depends to an enormous degree on the comparisons they make between themselves and others' (Tiefer 2004: 12). So when a woman breastfeeding a 4-year-old talks about 'being normal' at an LLL meeting, she means that she is 'normal' in a cultural-statistical sense, given her immediate surroundings – but this status alters in relation to her surroundings, for she is certainly not perceived as normal in wider society.

Tiefer makes the point that a person works out 'how I am doing' through a process of social comparison, not only by some internal standard. Exposure to a broad range of weaning ages means that what is 'normal' can be vastly stretched, even as it retains its symbolic power. One woman talked about her own horizons being widened by seeing a friend breastfeed her 8-year-old (whilst also recognising that there are limits to what 'normal' might be):

Charlotte: Have you ever seen anything at LLL that made you raise your eyebrows?

Ivana [*Leader applicant, 38, breastfeeding her 3-year-old daughter*]: I guess the longest that I have seen is [my friend] at 7 or 8, and I really, I didn't feel like raising an eyebrow, I thought wow! I felt quite inspired, not in the sense that I am going to do the same with [my child], necessarily, because it is up to her, but inspired that somebody is standing up in the way she did it, the way she followed her children and accommodated what they wanted. And very often mothers who breastfeed their children to 4 or 5 ... at least some of them get very sort of tired, and feel they should stop because of the social pressures, which I thought, on one side I understand, but on the other side I think that really [it's good to have that inspiration] ... if it was a 13-year-old or something, I don't know.

In a society where it is unusual to see a baby being breastfed, seeing women at LLL meetings breastfeeding children who walk and talk can be quite a surprise:

Pippa [*Long-serving leader*]: … it was actually my first LLL meeting. And there was this mum there who was about five months pregnant, and she had this toddler there with her who was very restless, and all of a sudden she just lifted her tee shirt and latched him on. And I thought, gosh, she is pregnant, and she can breastfeed! And a baby that big too. It didn't raise my eyebrows, it just opened my eyes. I was surprised, but I wasn't shocked, or outraged or anything.

Seeing women breastfeed toddlers, breastfeed twins, breastfeed whilst pregnant or breastfeed up to four children were only some of the things women said had surprised them.

Norms

To describe collective expectations for the proper behaviour of actors with a given identity is to describe 'norms'. Norms are not just statistical reflections: they have a potentiality in the sense that they engender certain, arguably coercive, effects. Indeed, the relationship between statistical and ideal norms is an iterative one. Andrews (1991) contends that LLL's philosophy acts as a form of social control. As Katzenstein has written, in some situations 'norms operate like rules that define the identity of an actor, thus having "constitutive effects" that specify what actions will cause relevant others to recognise a particular identity' (Katzenstein 1966: 5, in Keck and Sikkink 1998: 3).

LLL meetings should be seen as a space where women can express their thoughts about mothering their children, free from the pressures of judgement typical of the outside world. As one woman said:

Jane [*Leader applicant, 25, breastfeeding her 16-month-old son*]: I did feel like everyone I know from LLL is my sort of person. You don't have to talk about things that you all do all the time. You all do this so you can talk about something else. You don't have to explain yourself, which gets really tiring!

Nevertheless, the meetings are – to use Goffman's term – a space of performance: 'I assume that when an individual appears before others he will have many motives for trying to control the impression they receive of the situation. … The issues dealt with by stage-craft and stage management are sometimes trivial but they are quite general; they seem to occur everywhere in social life, providing a clear-cut dimension for sociological analysis' (Goffman 1959: 26). To say that mothers perform motherhood is not to imply that it is a mask under which they keep their 'real' selves; rather, it is part of a mother's self-making, or identity work (Murphy 1999). Women at LLL meetings are very conscious of being a mother amongst an audience of mothers – that is, after all, why they have come.[1] The vast majority of women spoke gratefully about finding the league, and about their relief at finding like-minded people to share experiences with and, frequently, socialise with in the local area outside of meetings. (This was particularly the case for women who had recently moved to the UK, for whom LLL offered a ready-made network.)

Yet I quickly realised how much certain norms become internalised, and operate as rules: having been to just two meetings, I had worked out that it was important to bring some sort of offering, and that it should be one that reflected a commitment to the LLL philosophy of eating foods in 'as close to their natural state as possible'. Because I was sometimes going to two meetings in a day, travelling across London, taking homemade cakes (my original plan) soon proved too difficult. Dried apricots became a staple, though I worried that people would think they did not reflect enough effort on my part, or that they were not generous enough or too full of sugar.

These 'norms' come to define group boundaries. Clarke's (2007) analysis of children's birthday parties shows how consumption patterns mark different mothers as inside and outside a particular group. She gives the example of a mother who 'exposes' the children to Smarties (a popular sweet) at a child's birthday party, which breaks a 'sacred, but unwritten, rule regarding the exposure of infants to impurities such as sugar' (Clarke 2007: 273), thereby putting the mother in an uncomfortable relationship to the other mothers. Judy said, about LLL:

> *Judy [39, breastfeeding her 2- and 4-year-old daughters]*: We didn't have problems breastfeeding, we had problems socialising. When you get to certain points, people want to roll out the parties and drinks and things, and when you go to an LLL event you find normal foods, like hummus and rice cakes and, when you go to an event outside the LLL community you find fairy cakes and sugary biscuits and juice drinks.

Engendering a sense of belonging (to a group) depends upon distinguishing an 'us' from a 'them' (Douglas 1986). Judy's comments do precisely this: LLL's values are represented in the food available at meetings, which differs from what would typically be available at other parent-child events. Other parents 'outside the LLL community' apparently do not have the same values about what children consume.

The coercive aspect of these norms was also evident. LLL says that it supports all mothers, though most women also noted that it would be a brave woman who came along and formula-fed her child (as part of mixed feeding), or who announced she would be weaning at 3 months old:

> *Charlotte*: Does LLL have the reputation of being extreme?
>
> *Leticia [36, 3½-year-old son, breastfeeding her 2-year-old daughter, emphasis added]*: Yes. ... And I think it is only partly true. Yeah, there are people in LLL who feed their kids until 4 or 5 or 6 and that is, in this society that is extreme, whether you like it or not. That is an extreme choice. And so, *even though the message is always, and they always repeat this at every meeting, you know, that there is no pressure to feed for any length of time, they really support anyone feeding for however long they want, but there is this expectation that you will feed for as long as you are physically capable,* and I don't mean in terms of the age, I mean in terms of let's say going back to work that you should really *try* as much as possible to breastfeed by expressing. So there is *a subtle pressure there to do your best to have a commitment to your child and to breastfeeding.* ... Which on many levels I support, because I do think that breastfeeding is the best thing for the child, and the best thing for the mother and the best thing for the mother and child together, I do support that, but I think, I have been in a situation where I have brought friends who are committed to breastfeeding, but maybe also needing other elements in their lives that don't necessarily fit with the people who go to LLL and I know they have felt excluded being there, and judged.

In fact, at one meeting, when one mother *did* announce she would be weaning (ceasing breastfeeding entirely) at 6 months so that she could go back to work, the room fell quiet. Eventually, a leader said, 'LLL has plenty to offer women considering weaning, though you may be interested to hear that a lot of women successfully manage to combine breastfeeding with working.' The mother did not come to the next month's meeting.[2]

Thus 'norms' act over time to shape women's perceptions. Accepting tenets of LLL's philosophy in the early months of a child's life – that babies should be breastfed on cue, for example – logically leads women to accept others, such as that children should also be breastfed 'to full term'. Both of these precepts hinge on belief in the efficacy of evolutionary narratives in explaining and determining biologically appropriate care for children, as discussed in the following chapter. To some extent the logic acts as a slippery slope, despite the fact that women are highly reflexive about their practices. Furthermore, because these mothers reflect on their practices amongst those who share a moral consensus about mothering, questions of what is 'normal' (i.e., natural, right, appropriate) become increasingly distinct from those found in wider society. A mother seeking support for breastfeeding her 6-month-old can find herself socialising with those who breastfeed far older children. As the rest of her friends outside the LLL community cease breastfeeding, she may be torn as to which network to ascribe to. LLL provides a set of norms by which to structure her identity work via one particular form of intensive mothering. It can be hard for women to bridge these norms, leading some mothers to 'only feel comfortable with my LLL friends' (Amelia).

La Leche League as Purposeful Network

The structure of LLL – a 'league' – as a purposeful network provides the framework for expression and maintenance of these 'norms' about mothering. For some of the women in the attachment mother group, then, this is not just a collection of individuals but, as Sally puts it, a social *movement* or 'a new way of parenting, which is post tribal, post industrial – and quite exciting to be part of'.

Wilkinson (1971) describes a social movement as a series of actions and endeavours of a body of persons for a special object (Wilkinson 1971). It is a 'deliberate and collective endeavour to promote change in any direction and by any means, not excluding violence, illegality, revolution or withdrawal into "utopian" community'. Some form of organisation is critical to this (e.g., the league network). What is most crucial, however, is commitment to change and the raison d'être of the organisation as founded upon the 'conscious volition, normative commitment to the movement's aims or beliefs, and active participation on the part of the followers or members' (Wilkinson 1971: 27).

Mothering, LLL philosophy reminds us, strengthens the very fabric of society – this is, arguably, the 'aim' of the movement for my informants, mediated via breastfeeding. It is a micro-practice that has impact on the macro scale, via a trickle-down effect. For Ginsburg and Rapp, an anthropological study of reproduction goes beyond a literal study of procreation, since children are always born into 'complex social arrangements through which legacies of property, positions, rights, and values are negotiated over time. [Therefore i]n its biological and social senses, it is inextricably bound up with the production of culture.... [b]y using reproduction as an entry point into the study of social life, we can see how cultures are produced (or contested) as people imagine and enable the creation of the next generation, most directly though the nurturance of children' (Ginsburg and Rapp 1995: 1–2).

This is social reproduction in the broadest sense then – of children, and of values:

> *Charlotte*: What is the point of 'loving guidance' [the LLL stance on how to discipline children]?
>
> *Liz* [*Long-serving leader*]: Well, it is about making humane humans, I suppose. And what does that mean? It means not being on your own at Christmas; it means relationships. The fabric of society is improved through good mothering ... it's about that solidarity, the caring.... It's about creating caring human beings.

In her article *Pregnancy and Infant Loss Support: A New, Feminist, American, Patient Movement?*, Layne (2006) argues that the support groups she studied might be understood as a social movement, in that they are an example of 'political organising around a common identity' (Layne 2006: 697, drawing on Taylor and Whittier 1992: 105). Yet some scholars, she points out, do not consider these groups social movements because the extent to which they wish to change society remains ambiguous, an observation applicable to this case as well: 'Critics of mutual-aid groups argue that they do not qualify as social movements because their agendas are personal, rather than political.... Similarly, critics of co-dependency support groups argue that such groups offer "a false sense of empowerment while taking energy away from political solutions to political problems"' (Layne 2006: 608, quoting Lodl in Irvine 1999: 130). La Leche League itself states unequivocally that as an organisation it is *apolitical*, by which it means it does not 'campaign' for changes at the societal level that would make following its philosophy more realisable (such as flexible work hours for mothers; see above).

Activism

Yet the language of empowerment and choice sits well within the feminist agenda to which many of the attachment mothers subscribe. Like others who were attracted to the organisation, one woman speaks of how LLL appealed to her own inclinations towards political engagement through awareness-raising:

> *Charlotte*: I met you at an LLL meeting – why did you come?
>
> *Gayle [32, breastfeeding her 8-month-old daughter]*: I found the idea quite appealing, politically I suppose, to be honest ... I just liked the idea of an organisation that campaigned for breastfeeding, and that disseminated accurate information about breastfeeding, and associated things about co-sleeping and all the rest of it. I mean, politically they sort of strike me as being slightly anarchist, which I quite like actually ... I think it was a deliberate political decision to get involved with what they are doing.

Certainly, some women I met enjoyed a deliberate political engagement through the LLL network, particularly when it came to the promotion of breastfeeding (not full-term breastfeeding per se, though it is notable that many women who do promote breastfeeding are also those who breastfeed to full term). The projection into society of their values is an important part of their identity work, in that it validates their own choices. Sandra, an LLL Leader, touched on this:

> *Charlotte*: How did you come to LLL?
>
> *Sandra [Leader, 35, breastfeeding her 4-year-old daughter]*: I had heard of them before I had her ... I read everything I could get my hands on about breastfeeding really.... And actually I had thought that they were much more of a protest, campaigning organisation. And I suppose I had that view of a militant organisation. Which, unlike a lot of other people, didn't put me off actually, unlike a lot of people, because I think, deep down in myself, when I'm being [me] and don't have my leader's hat on, I am quite militant about it.

In line with some of the more campaign-style activities this leader describes, a public 'nurse-in'[3] was organised during the fieldwork as part of Breastfeeding Awareness Week (Figure 5.1; note that many women are breastfeeding older children, including the 3-year-old boy walking around at the front).[4]

Resistance

As Layne's case indicates, it is hard to say whether women's full-term breastfeeding and attachment parenting is a form of 'activism', given that mothering in this way is largely the adoption of a position

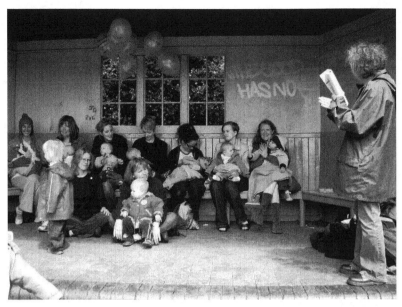

FIGURE 5.1. A 'nurse-in,' London, May 2006, author's photo

of *resistance*. Women resist 'the mainstream' through quiet acts of rebellion (see also Bobel 2002; Scott 1995), meaning that for many of them, literally 'everything they do is political' (Virginia).[5] This is not the politics of running for office or of grand social change, but rather a means of political engagement through daily interactions within communities and families. As in the feminist movement of the 1970s, with which LLL has some congruence, 'the personal is political'.

This was evident in numerous areas of women's lives. Perhaps the most obvious site of 'resistance to culture' is mothers' work. Most of the breastfeeding women in my sample commented that they were 'lucky' to be able to mother as they did. Only one mother in the group of twenty-five UK women said in the questionnaire that she was working full-time (eight said they worked part-time, and four that they were on maternity leave; the remaining twelve were not working). Many said they were living 'simply' so they could spend time with their children, sacrificing what they saw as the trappings of consumer culture to do so (fashionable clothes, holidays, expensive houses and cars, etc). Yet it was clear that they were able to 'choose' to live simply, rather than having it forced upon them through poverty. A secure financial base and a high educational and class status meant they could afford to take risks others cannot.

Work was generally understood to be a dehumanising experience. Working for money was seen as important for some people
– but these mothers had 'made the decision' to be at home with
their children. This decision was therefore a way of distancing oneself from 'other mothers'. As Bobel puts it, women who go to work
are often perceived to be supporting their own materialism, not doing so because of any real 'need', as Jane indicated:

> *Jane* [*Leader applicant, 25, breastfeeding her 16-month-old son*]: I think if
> people did understand the philosophy they wouldn't go back to work,
> even if they didn't have very much money. I mean, I don't think peo-
> ple need to work.... I mean some people feel they need to, [but] you
> can actually manage on less than you think.[6]

Women therefore constituted themselves as different from the
norm. They had not always planned to do this, however – as discussed
later, this was part of an 'enlightenment process' they underwent:

> *Jemima* [*Chair of Council, emphasis added*]: It was just amazing to find
> people who really did have similar thoughts to how I had been think-
> ing.... I was an investment banker so my rational mind would have
> told me to go back to the City and earn a fortune, but *the mothering
> even took over my life really....* So yeah, I sort of had *this light bulb mo-
> ment where I realised that the most important thing in this planet was to be
> mother to these children,* and not run [the bank].

In this view, the world of work (and investment banking in particular) cannot be compared to what it means to be a mother. The
difference is not one of degree, but one of kind. There is no job on
the planet more important than raising children. Another woman's
questionnaire response indicated the extent to which mothering
had become her source of identity work:

> *Questionnaire*: What does it mean to be a mother?
>
> *Valerie* [*33, breastfeeding her 11-month-old son*]: It means everything
> to me and defines who I am now. Career and money are no longer
> the life goal, my child and future family happiness are my focus and
> source of pride and success.

The very definition of intimate social relations places them in opposition to the world of commerce (Miller 1997; Zelizer 1985). Con-
sumerism fuels the capitalist economy that depends increasingly on
mothers working outside the home, so 'when a mother refuses to
"buy into" the notion that her worth is established by a paycheck or

a job title, she performs an act of resistance.... The natural mother not only asserts herself as the 'naturally best' caretaker of her children, but consciously withdraws from a segment of consumer culture' (Bobel 2002: 119–120).

Removing oneself from the spend-work-spend cycle is considered a political act (Bobel 2002: 120). As a lifestyle, simplified living was therefore a form of activism: using leftovers, making one's own clothes, growing one's own vegetables. And for some women, their desire not to work was tied to their rejection of institutionalised childcare:

> *Chloe* [*Long-serving anglophone leader*]: I went in [to the nursery] one day, just because I was worried about him ... [and] once, John was asleep and there was a baby crying and they were on their lunch or something, and just letting it cry horribly, at you know 3 months old. And finally I picked it up and consoled it just because I couldn't stand it.... I thought, that could be John, and they will just let him cry!

The criticism of childcare frequently extended to other sorts of formal education, which are seen as putting rational institutional measurement above individual needs. Amongst the group of mothers I interviewed, homeschooling was more prevalent than amongst the average UK population (4 out of the 22 women were homeschooling, or intending to homeschool).[7]

Conclusion

This chapter has shown how La Leche League offers people a framework within which to account for, legitimate and celebrate their non-conventional mothering. LLL engenders a sense of belonging for its members: it is not simply an informal network of people, but a formalised organisation. It offers a framework in which motherhood can be turned into a career, and not only in the sense that women are encouraged to perform identity work through their mothering: they can also achieve badges of professionalisation by becoming 'leaders' and district leaders, and by sitting on the board of directors or even on international committees.

The analysis now turns to how women practising full-term breastfeeding account for their non-normative practices as part of their identity work. Many of their accountability strategies – which rely on recourse to evolution, nature, science and feeling – are presented and discussed at LLL meetings.

Notes

1. There was a twist, however, in how mothers negotiated these performances, in that they were *projected* performances. Children's behaviour at meetings was read as a marker of their mothers' own capacities, echoing my argument here. Women would not be frowned upon if children were crying, or causing havoc, for example – rather, a deliberate attempt would be made to reassure the mother that it was not a problem, with the aim of fostering a welcoming atmosphere. But mothers themselves certainly internalised the sense of audience. Women would apologise if their child crashed into me as we sat on the floor, or was screaming loudly in my ear. To be sure, this is not specific to LLL meetings, but rather a comment on a more pervasive climate of intensive motherhood where 'we are all monitoring each other', as one interviewee put it (see Chapter 1).

2. It is interesting that questions of accountability operate at both ends of the infant feeding spectrum: where Lee reports in her work with formula feeding mothers a sense of stigmatisation and need to offer explanations for 'deviance' (2008), a mother who had recently stopped breastfeeding her 4-year-old son felt the need to explain that 'I would have let him go on, but it was his decision.'

3. This photo was taken at a public protest where numerous members of the press were present.

4. This annual week, dedicated to raising awareness about breastfeeding in the UK, has been run by the Department of Health since 1993 and is supported by many lay organisations (LLL, NCT, Association of Breastfeeding Mothers, etc). Again, this highlights the congruence between lay organisations and the state.

5. It is interesting that although many women constitute themselves as going 'against the grain' of mainstream care practices, attachment parenting is implicitly advocated by a range of (governmental) agencies today: for instance, practices such as long-term, on-demand breastfeeding and skin-to-skin contact are widely advocated by the Department of Health.

6. This subject revealed some intra-group fault lines. Some mothers who confided in me in private spoke about their resentment of the mothers who had the resources to mother as they themselves would like to do and made them feel guilty for not 'trying harder':

   Wendy [35, breastfeeding her 2-year-old son]: I mean, you are made to feel a bit bad sometimes. You know, I had to put my son in the nursery, because I needed to work. I am a single mum. And some people do make you feel a bit guilty about that. And you think, 'You have no idea – this is really hard for me.'

7. Between 20,000 and 40,000 children aged 5–16 are estimated to be educated at home in the UK. According to the 1996 education act in England and Wales, it is parents who are responsible for providing their children with education, 'in school or otherwise', suitable for the age, ability and aptitude of each child. The same provision is not made in France.

Part III

ACCOUNTING FOR FULL-TERM BREASTFEEDING

Chapter 6

'It's Natural'
Some Cultural Contradictions

What anthropologists say: Determining what is a natural age of weaning for human beings raises some problems. *Human beings' ideas about when and how to wean are often determined by culture, not necessarily by what is best or natural for babies and mothers.* Anthropologists who have studied weaning have found a great variety in weaning ages, from birth (in much of the United States and Western society in general) to age seven or eight in other cultures.... Dr Dettwyler has used the example of primates to try to determine a natural weaning age for humans, since 'gorillas and chimpanzees share more than ninety-eight percent of their genes with humans' but are *lacking the cultural biases* of humans.

—D. Bengson, *How Weaning Happens* (emphasis added)

B reastfeeding to full term – anything between one and eight years in this study, though more typically for three or four years – is considered by attachment mothers to be part of a 'natural' trajectory, doing justice to a hominid blueprint for behaviour. The blueprint is derived from archaeological and anthropological evidence of humans as primates, in some cases through historical studies of our evolutionary past, and in others through recourse to contemporary primates or 'primitive' peoples who are understood to represent that past today.

Yet being natural is a profoundly cultural process (Strathern 1992b), especially where women following the LLL philosophy of breastfeeding until the child 'outgrows the need' constitute themselves as marginal with respect to mainstream patterns of care.

Women mobilise the moral authority of the natural to explain, justify and 'account' for their non-conventional parenting practices, and specifically their long-term breastfeeding. The 'natural' to which women refer is multiple and elastic: known internally through 'gut feelings', revealed through 'scientific findings' and validated by the 'evolutionary' narratives focused on in this chapter. Indeed, the natural is the thread running through each of the accountability strategies, addressed in turn. For those who wish to ground their moral vision in external reality, the attraction of nature is arguably its capacity to make disputed values seem innate, essential, eternal and non-negotiable (Wall 2001).

Women's accounts of doing what is 'most natural' are framed as a form of 'cultural contradiction' (Hays 1996) in this chapter, which offers both a description and critique of women's reference to primitives and primates. (To this extent it draws on Hausman's work on this subject [2003: chapter 5, passim]). The character of women's feminism is explored by examining the role of fathers in attachment parenting and the contradiction between paternal involvement and body-based discourses of natural (maternal) embodied care. The double lens of the anthropologist – participating in, yet objectifying, social life – is particularly relevant in working with people who rely on dichotomies (such as nature/culture) fundamental to the discipline itself.

Types of Natural: Some Accounts

A rhetoric of the natural is a major accountability strategy in women's narratives of full-term breastfeeding. Ivana and Megan are quoted at length here because their answers encompass many of the themes articulated by others:

> *Charlotte*: Can you give me three reasons why you wanted to breastfeed, and why you are still breastfeeding?
>
> *Ivana* [*Leader applicant, 38, breastfeeding her 3-year-old daughter, emphasis added*]: Only three? … we always discuss this sort of thing. I think there are *social* reasons, *health* reasons – physical, emotional, psychological … and the third one, *political* reasons I guess. On a physical health reason, there are a lot of things that are good for the baby and the mother…. But those are, I mean, of course health is important, but I think breastfeeding, for me, almost more important, is experiencing how breastfeeding fulfils so many needs of the baby, especially the newborn, and how it does it in such a perfect way. [To not use]

what is given for free, for the best possible nourishment in so many levels, it is almost like a wasting of a resource ... wasting the gift, wasting the opportunities ... *I think it is a bit arrogant towards nature.* It is also linked to the political level. ... Not supporting the world, the planet, the earth ... just something you can exploit for your benefit and discard ... and so it is better to use it in a rational maximising sort of way. A very simple example would be formula, to produce it you need so much input, you need the cows, you need to farm them, transport it, to condense it, which takes resources, you have to package it, you have to sell it, you have to throw away the packaging, and plus it is not perfect for the human baby. ... And on the other side you have something which is just there, which is perfect. So yeah, that is one reason.

[*Later Ivana said, in terms of social reasons*]: I feel generations of people born in the fifties, sixties, seventies, eighties, I think there was an impact from non-breastfeeding practices ... and I think a lot of the problems that we have are linked to that, not just to pollution and all that stuff. I don't know; the atomisation of society, the disconnection.

Megan [41, breastfeeding her 4-year-old son, emphasis added]: You see, the thing is Charlotte, what I'm doing *is* normal – you know, it's actually *the most natural thing in the world* when you think about it. Children have a *need* for their mother's milk until the age of six, and mothers are designed to fulfil that need. *It feels right, because it's part of our evolution.* The benefits are in the literature. The people who have a problem with it just don't realise what they're saying. If they did, they would see that this is, this is ... it's liquid gold we're talking about here, you know ... their trouble is that they can't see past the method of delivery. *In lots of tribal societies women breastfeed for this long,* and it's just not an issue for them.

When women talk about their decision to continue breastfeeding their children, they evoke nature in two general ways. In one sense, they refer to the inherent force that directs the world, or human beings – or both. In the other, they refer to the material world itself, which in some cases includes human beings but at other times does not (Williams 1988: 219). Within this double evocation lie clear contradictions. 'Culture' is envisaged as an ingredient adding refinement to a shared 'animal nature', but at the same time it is human nature to create culture. Women can therefore look to nature for justification of extended breastfeeding (in 'tribal societies') and at the same time validate it as something they 'feel' is right (as in, natural). The internal/external duality takes a final twist: in the case of these mothers, 'being natural' is enacted on the grounds of strengthening culture, since stronger bonds between mothers and children

– the end product of the LLL philosophy – are understood to repair the damaged fabric of society.[1]

For many women, the child itself *is* nature, embodied in a pure form at birth and expressed in the belief that a baby's natural development should not be interfered with – that is, that children should be breastfed 'on cue' as well as 'until they outgrow the need'. As Miller comments, on the basis of his work with mothers in London: 'All demands express [the child's] purity as nature, which should be immediately met' (Miller 1997: 74). This is evident in the way women talk about not only the 'natural course' of child development, but also the feeding of children exclusively with breast milk as a means to preserve their organic status – breast milk is nature's 'perfect food', says Ivana.

Miller notes that parents understand a child's development as a series of defeats, as they attempt to protect them against the damaging influences of the external, artificial world. Judy recounted her disgust that the hospital staff had given her baby a bottle of formula milk rather than her expressed breast milk: 'to think that they lined her stomach with that poison was so upsetting', she said. The drive to protect their children's purity from infection by the outside world was manifest at all ages. The LLL philosophy specifies whole, organic, home-made foods 'in as close to their natural state as possible' as ideal. Many mothers here saw processed or 'junk' foods as artificial pollutants, and much anxiety surrounded their consumption. One leader spoke of her shame at having served shop-bought cakes at her first monthly meeting because her dog had eaten the fruit loaf she made that morning.

To quote Wall, 'On one level, then, breast milk, given its status as a natural substance, as opposed to an artificial one, is understood to be essentially, and unquestionably, pure and good. The possibility that nature is not always a positive force and that natural substances also can be less than pure is left unaddressed' (2001: 596–597). 'Natural' is a concept around which strong feelings can coalesce, but actual practices remain unspecified. It is the elasticity of the concept – the stretching and contracting to be at once normal, right, non-artificial, traditional, instinctive – that makes it so powerful in women's accountability strategies, and so fundamental to their identity work.

Natural Parenting

Fashions in parenting are best understood as barometers of wider cultural trends, which recently have seen a growing validation of the 'natural' way to do things as diverse as eating, learning and treating illness. This stance rests on an enduring conviction that nature is a force to be trusted and respected; regarding parenting, it advocates deference to the 'natural' bond between mother and child (paraphrased from Bobel 2002: 11). Felicity, for example, alludes to these beliefs:

> Felicity [33, 12-year-old daughter, just-weaned 2-year-old son]: I believe in clean natural living ... formula is like feeding your kids vitamin-fortified McDonalds happy meals ... convenient yes, looks like real food, but isn't real food. I have respect for nature and the one million years it's taken to perfect breast milk ... I owe it to them to do right by them to the best of my ability.

For attachment mothers, resisting nature – by not breastfeeding at all or not breastfeeding for as long as the child has a need – is dangerous. Ivana sees it as being 'arrogant' towards nature. Felicity 'owes it to her children' to 'respect' the processes of evolution. Modern culture is seen to be eroding humanity's proper place on the planet. The women's accounts are therefore a profound statement about the place of humans within the cosmological order, at once radical (in the sense of wanting to create social change) and conservative (in the sense of wanting to return to a prior, premodern state).

Full-term breastfeeding is but one choice women make in cultivating a natural lifestyle – many (though not all) attachment mothers follow the same logic in other areas of their lives. They often favoured the rhythm method of contraception over pills or intrauterine devices, which were understood to disrupt the body's natural state. When they had their period, they did not use tampons or sanitary towels but a 'menstrual cup', which was more environmentally friendly. At birth they would eschew interventions and avoid painkillers where possible. Women often used cloth nappies for their children, which were said to be better for the environment (though some women countered that the detergents used to wash them were just as harmful). Children were not necessarily vaccinated, and medical treatments for illness, such as antibiotics, were used only as a last resort, as they were held to interrupt the body's own homeostasis. The family would eat primarily organic, local, whole foods if they could. They abstained from wearing synthetic or branded clothes whenever possible. They recycled. They preferred cycling to driving, and making their own food rather than buying it. As Bobel puts it, long-term breastfeeding women resist culture to embrace nature in almost all areas of their lives (Bobel 2002: 125; also see Chapter 5).

The use of nature to advocate particular forms of behaviour is nothing new. Rousseau is one famous case in point:

> Do you want to bring everyone back to his first duties? Begin with mothers. You will be surprised by the changes you will produce. Everything follows successively from this first depravity [wet-nursing]. The whole moral order degenerates; naturalness is extinguished in all hearts; the toughening spectacle of the family aborning no longer attaches husbands, no longer imposes respect on outsiders.... There are no longer fathers, mothers, children, brothers or sisters. They hardly know each other. How could they love each other? But let mothers deign to nurse their children, morals will reform themselves, nature's sentiments will be awakened in every heart, the state will be repopulated. (Rousseau 1979 [1762]: 46, in Kukla 2005: 30)

Yet this 'looking to nature', as a trend that has become particularly prominent in recent years, is worthy of a closer look. Unconfined to marginal social networks, it is ever more prominent in policy, which relies increasingly on evolutionary narratives in recommendations of appropriate infant care. Infant sleep is one good example (Ball 2007).[2] Ball advocates the practice of bed-sharing, stating at the 2006 LLLGB conference, for example, that the practice of putting infants to sleep in a separate bed was 'historically novel, culturally circumscribed, developmentally inappropriate and evolutionarily bizarre'. Her argument is that in comparison to other primates, human infants are drastically more neurologically immature at birth due to the play-off between being big-brained and being bipedal (which requires birthing through a narrow pelvis). Human infants therefore require more intensive care than other primate infants (constant bodily contact to regulate heat, for example).

To argue that human beings do not have evolutionary adaptations or expectations (e.g., of food to eat), or that these are not particularly acute in infancy, would of course be foolish. What is of interest here is the point at which 'expectations' – which some parents will no doubt find reassuring – become injunctions (some enshrouded in policy) in the form of parenting practices carried out over many years. There are often moral messages behind arguments for certain styles of care, particularly those that endorse long-term embodied care by the mother. The operation of the natural as a domain of foundational cultural practice has always been a site of anthropological interest, and recent years have seen the birth of a tradition that foregrounds the 'constitutive role of metaphor, analogy, classification, narrative, and genealogy in the production of natural facts' (Franklin 1990: 127) – a tradition engaged with here.

Evolutionary Narratives: Primates and 'Primitives'

It is typical to hear attachment mothers, such as Megan, account for the decision to breastfeed to full term in the language of evolutionary adaptation and development. In lay terms, the idea is that women should breastfeed the way primates and primitive humans did (or do), since our bodies adapted to a specific form of lactation because it was evolutionarily advantageous (Hausman 2003).

Many of the women I worked with referred to *Our Babies, Ourselves* (Small 1998), a text that takes an evolutionary perspective to rationalise particular parenting techniques. According to Small, breasts probably evolved as an adaptive feature of small, egg-laying animals that populated the earth in the period following the extinction of the dinosaurs (the Mesozoic).[3] This species would keep their eggs warm by sitting on them, at the same time nourishing them by secreting a fluid rich in antibacterial lysosome. When the eggs hatched, the infants probably licked some of this coating, which became immunologically protective on ingestion. Those that licked the most fluid accrued the most advantages in terms of growth, and therefore those mothers with the most abundant secretions were selected for (Small 1998: 181).

The first mammary gland, Small postulates, was probably something like a sweat gland that excreted substance from the inside of the body to the outside. 'Eventually these chest glands changed into apocrine glands, tissue that can synthesise proteins, carbohydrates, and lipids, rather than just excrete water' (Small 1998: 181). This evolution occurred in tandem with the infant's ability to suckle. Mammals were characterised by a high level of investment in offspring kept close at hand, nourished by a fluid produced in the female body.[4] The female's ability to consume a range of foods (not suitable for infants) and process them into a single fluid that could sustain life for a considerable period of time was highly adaptive. In species where mothers feed their infants infrequently (and leave them in the nest for long periods of time), milk is high in fat and protein, so the infants remain satisfied longer. Human infants fed breast milk, which is low in fat and protein, require more regular feeding, says Small.

The mothers interviewed here also widely cited the biological anthropologist Katherine Dettwyler when they used this particular accountability strategy. She uses cross-cultural, cross-species and cross-temporal examples of a range of factors, including age of eruption of first molar and length of gestation, to come to a blueprint for human weaning, free of 'culture':

The primary purpose of this chapter is to attempt to answer one specific question: At what age would human infants be weaned (cease
breastfeeding completely) if the process were based only on physiological considerations? That is, acknowledging that humans are
primates, and recognizing that lactation and weaning take place according to certain patterns in non-human primates, then what do
these patterns suggest would be the natural age of weaning in modern
humans if these behaviours were not modified by culture? (Dettwyler
1995: 39)

Dettwyler concludes:

[I]f humans weaned their offspring according to the primate pattern
without regard to beliefs and customs, most children would be weaned
somewhere between 2.5 and 7 years of age. (Dettwyler 1995: 66)

It was sometimes difficult, as a social anthropologist, to explain to
mothers that not all of 'what anthropologists say' translates into an
advocacy perspective (whether from the biological or social perspective). The use of anthropological research by non-anthropologists
certainly poses some interesting ethical questions for the ethnographer, particularly if any confusion as to what 'sort' of anthropologist
one is exists at the point of data collection – that is, if it influences
people's willingness to share accounts, on the basis of the perceived
ends of the research. Clifford and Marcus (1986) note that increasingly, ethnographers all over the world must contend with the use
of anthropological evidence by their subjects of research. Indeed,
this proved a difficult issue during this project: in Dettwyler's narrative, nature is something monolithic, distinct, unsullied by culture
and best represented by primates living 'in the wild' (Bobel 2002:
127). But as Hausman (2003) notes, that humans could ever be cul-
ture-free is quite a startling assertion for an anthropologist to make,
even in the name of an exercise.

Primates

Donna Haraway has described the field of primatology as a cultural
landscape. Primates acquire a special status, she argues, as 'natural
objects that can show people their origin, and therefore their prera-
tional, premanagement, precultural essence … [providing] the point
of union of the physiological and political for modern liberal theo-
rists while they continue to accept the ideology of the split between
nature and culture' (Haraway 1978a: 26).

A cross-species blueprint for the time of weaning assumes no interaction between animal and environment – or culture – which,

as many primatologists will argue, is not, and has never been, the case: 'Primate infant nutrition is strongly influenced by the ecological and social environment, generating the hypothesis that *flexibility characterising the process is adaptive,* allowing individual organisms to improve the fit between themselves and their local environment' (Wells 2006: 45, emphasis added). In other words, whilst some primates *might* wean their offspring at a very late age where suitable weaning foods do not exist, this is not necessarily the case where resources are more bountiful. Indeed, where weaning foods are readily available, primate behaviour is characterised by decreased length of lactation to enable the mother to invest her labours in gestating and nurturing other offspring (Wells 2006).

Furthermore, active weaning behaviour is a feature common to almost all mammals. The comparative zoologist Trivers (1974) was the first to propose this, in his 'Parent-Offspring Conflict' thesis. His argument was that there was a conflict between a mother's urge to reproduce and pass on her genes, and her infant's desire to benefit as much as possible from maternal care (in turn to survive and reproduce). This is usually mediated in degrees as the infant matures, eventually culminating with the mother adopting quite fierce weaning tactics, such as biting or kicking her infant (Blaffer Hrdy 2000). (Indeed, a range of authors have problematised the relevance of primate studies for our understandings of human behaviour, particularly Eyer in her book *Mother-Infant Bonding: A Scientific Fiction* [1992]. She argues against the concept of a bonding 'window', witnessed in some animals during the immediate postnatal period and often referred to by attachment parenting advocates to stress the importance of skin-to-skin contact after birth [and in the early years]. Instead, it seems likely that in language-using mammals, *flexibility* in the process of relating would be adaptive.)

Primitives

The idea that humans essentially have the same body today as they did 400,000 years ago is, for many women, a way to rationalise 'full-term' breastfeeding. The environmental conditions under which early humans lived shaped their physiology and their biosocial practices: danger from predators (meaning a need to have infants close at hand so as to stifle any loud cry, usually by nursing); a lack of appropriate weaning foods (meaning prolonged breastfeeding); and a continuous cycle of pregnancy and lactation for fertile females, during which prolonged lactation helped space childbirth at optimal intervals for infant survival (paraphrased from Hausman 2003: 128).

Mapping this blueprint onto contemporary circumstances means our biology has become a problem. According to attachment mothers, norms of modern infant care (perceived to be at the 'structured' end of the spectrum) such as scheduled sleeping and feeding routines are 'out of sync' with the evolutionary requirements of human beings. Part of the appeal of attachment mothering is that the model is imitative of infant care practices following an ancestral pattern that is biologically appropriate to the human species – that is, not only traditional, but *adaptive* in a biological sense (Hausman 2003: 124–125). This is a very powerful notion: 'The idea that specific, supposedly traditional, mothering practices are really evolutionary adaptations – rather than cultural constructions that emerge at a specific historical juncture – is a persuasive rhetoric, delineating natural and unnatural maternal practices within a speculative evolutionary paradigm' (Hausman 2003: 125). As part of attentive mothering, therefore, extended breastfeeding is appropriate to a child's need for emotional and physical support. Child-led weaning is 'natural,' whereas mother-led weaning is 'cultural' and therefore not appropriately biological (Hausman 2003: 125). Appropriate mothering in this framework is defined by the mother's ability to allow this evolutionary heritage to be expressed, which, despite the rhetoric of coming 'naturally,' can be an intensive, demanding task.

Typically, *contemporary* foraging societies are used as stand-ins for earlier hominid hunter-gatherers to represent 'natural' patterns of lactation and care, and statistics on length and frequency of lactation amongst them are used to demonstrate the ancestral pattern.[5] In the mid 1970s, Jean Liedloff, a self-trained anthropologist, aimed to re-introduce a style of 'traditional' parenting to the 'modern' world (see Bobel [2002: 61] for an account of this). Written on the basis of her time with the Yequana of Venezuela, *The Continuum Concept* method of childcare expounds a 'chain of experience of our species which is suited to the tendencies and expectations which we have evolved' (Liedloff 1985: 22–23). According to the continuum concept, babies are parented in the same way as those Liedloff witnessed in South America – they are held constantly by the mother or another close relative, are nursed on demand and sleep with the mother.

Using the example of the !Kung (an anthropological favourite – see Shostak 1981), Blaffer Hrdy has provided a critique of evolutionary theory and references to hunter-gatherers as used in the context of contemporary infant care. She argues that whilst the 'Environment of Evolutionary Adaptedness' – the millions of years during which today's humans' behavioural equipment would have evolved – is a useful theory, it has been sidelined to refer only to the Pleistocene period (see Hausman [2003: 143] for an account of this). Since most people assume that modern humans were, at one point, hunters on the African savannas, the !Kung of the Kalahari come to represent all hunter-gatherer peoples, and therefore, all peoples. This assumes a constancy of resources over time and space for all humans: '[The] extended half-decade of physical closeness between a mother and her infant [supposedly typified by the !Kung] … tells us more about the harshness of local conditions and the mothers' lack of safe alternatives than the "natural state" of *all* Pleistocene mothers' (Blaffer Hrdy 2000: 100–101). Local cultural traditions are largely ignored, and the !Kung (or the Yequana) are treated as passively representative of human biological patterns. They do not therefore act to create a culture of their own (the idea is that they *don't* have culture); rather, they stand in a vacuum (Hausman 2003: 143). To quote Wagner, in this 'search for origins',

> we run the grave risk of degenerating into a phrenology of brow ridges, foreheads, and cranial vaults, a fetishism of 'primitive' and 'animal-like' as opposed to 'progressive' and 'man like' details. Man is of course no less 'natural', no less of an animal, now than he has ever been. He is no more 'cultural' in his present state than his forebears were. (Wagner 1981: 137)

For Latour too, it is deeply political to envisage culture as something within which actors participate, as the act that separates us from other animals. To assume that the human ability to step outside culture and separate object from subject is what makes us 'modern' casts those that do not do so (primates and 'primitives') as acultural and therefore ahistorical. His argument is that we have 'never been modern', since we occupy a world where culture has never been separate from nature (Latour 1993).

The attachment mothers I worked with constructed 'the primitive' as a site for playing out fantasies of the natural: that !Kung wean their children by pasting bitter herbs onto their breasts (Small 1998: 82), or that they use enemas on their infants, both of which would likely be considered dangerous by attachment parents, is overlooked. A set of 'cultural blinkers' operates in mothers' attempts to emulate natural patterns of lactation (Buskens 2001).

The mothers I spoke with do not actually want the hunter-gatherer lifestyle, of course; rather, what we all wish to select are those elements that fit with our sensibilities. These mothers do not reject all forms of 'culture' – they retain the Internet, for example – but cultivate particular elements of 'nature' as part of the identity work that validates their mothering. Shostak's disappointment at not being able to emulate !Kung practice in her own breastfeeding, cut short by emergency surgery for breast cancer (Shostak 2000, cited in Hausman 2003), is highly problematic when one considers that the surgery available to her probably saved her life. To assume that, given the real possibility, !Kung mothers would not also have surgery or use painkillers in childbirth or formula milk for weaning is to ignore the evidence of numerous other societies. As soon as agriculture made soft weaning foods more available, weaning occurred earlier and babies were spaced more closely together (Blaffer Hrdy 2000: 201–202; Maher 1992; Palmer 1993). Human adaptation to local environments moves in a steady direction away from !Kung patterns of infant feeding, child care and fertility, which are extreme because of the harsh conditions under which the !Kung live.[6]

It is one thing, then, for a !Kung mother living where suitable weaning foods do not exist to breastfeed her 4-year-old, and quite a different thing for a woman living in London – and neither of them is more 'natural' than the other. A view of culture as something external to nature presents a dichotomy in which human interaction with, and manipulation of, the environment is considered artificial. Arguably, this adaptation – finding the best fit – is what evolution has always been about. What is notable amongst my informants is the particular way in which 'nature' is constructed as part of a cultural environment.

'Natural' Mothering: Feminism and Fathers

Bobel has argued that one of the most serious repercussions of the embodied mothering advocated by attachment parents is its marginalisation of fathers (Bobel 2002: 133). She notes that in her own study with 'natural' mothers in the US who also practise an attachment parenting philosophy, the division of labour falls along traditional lines, with women taking almost the entire responsibility for childcare.[7]

My informants generally described fathers as 'supportive'. Fathers in the more 'hard-core' couples in the group were actively involved in discussions of attachment parenting – about, for example, the merits of a family bed. Many women also mentioned how grateful they were for their husband's support during the early months of breastfeeding. Yet it seemed on the whole that fathers were accorded a passive role – they 'agreed' to share the bed with the child, and 'supported' the idea of full-term breastfeeding. One wonders whether they would have had strong objections if the mother had decided to put the baby in a separate room, formula feed, use a pushchair and so on. (The extent to which a father can insist that his partner breastfeed their child is, of course, an interesting question; certainly some women feel under pressure to feed in particular ways, for particular lengths of time. How families and couples go about making, and sticking to, their childcare decisions is clearly a complex issue.)

Many women mentioned that fathers would like to spend more time with their children but that 'sadly one of us has to bring home the bacon' (Virginia). In all cases it was typical that the father acted as primary breadwinner, rendering the mother responsible for the everyday embodied care of the child. This was usually narrated as common sense, or 'natural', particularly in the early months, because women understand themselves to be designed for mothering, with wombs, breasts and 'instincts' induced by the 'hormone of love' oxytocin:

> Megan [41, breastfeeding her 4-year-old son, emphasis]: I remember when he was born and started breastfeeding, and I did remember in relation to my breasts – because of our society and the culture we are in, and that sort of thing – thinking oh my god, that is what they are for.... And so it wasn't so much that I was wandering into the realms of extended breastfeeding, but more that, this is what I am designed for; to mother this baby. This is what I am programmed to feel and to do. You know, it feels natural, and there's a reason it feels natural. That was the biggest stone that dropped really, yeah. It was amazing, not to know now I look back.... Those first three days in the hospital. You know, to realise what they are for.

To quote Bobel: 'Roles flow from bodies in this view. According to the natural mothers, humans are pre-destined to act out certain roles as dictated by the structure and function of the biological bodily process' (Bobel 2002: 87). LLL shares this view:

> After birth, the intimate relationship between and mother and baby continues. They are still a unit, and for some time the mother will be the baby's sole source of nourishment. In a language that is irrefutable, biology makes it clear that the mother-baby relationship is primary and should not be set aside. This relationship is unique and sets the prototype for other relationships throughout life. A father's contribution is equally important, but is different. Babies thrive on both. (LLLI 2004: 185, emphasis added)

So fathers are important, but they do not have the same 'irrefutable biology'. LLL's philosophy continues: 'Breastfeeding is enhanced and the nursing couple sustained by the loving support, help, and companionship of the baby's father. A father's unique relationship with his baby is an important element in the child's development from early infancy.'[8]

A topic that came up frequently in LLL meetings, and to which a section is dedicated in the LLL book *The Womanly Art of Breastfeeding,* is the 'Manly Art of Fathering'. These discussions stress the importance of other jobs a father (or partner) can do to help with child-care, centring around protecting the mother-infant dyad and the breastfeeding relationship by offering to undertake other domestic chores, such as cleaning or cooking.[9] At none of the meetings I attended did the women approve of expressing breast milk to enable the father to take part in feeding (except as a last resort). Other tasks (such as bathing or changing) were said to be just as rewarding and intimate – though it is notable that in discussing these practices, 'bonding' was never talked about in the same way feeding was. One mother (not an attachment mother) said:

> Sunanda [*31, breastfeeding her 2-month-old son*]: My husband really feels he is missing out on the feeding … he has said that he really wants to feed him with a bottle at six months. So we are both at the point of 'what is good for him' and 'what is good for me' and you know, he said, he said it out loud, that he feels he is missing out, giving him something very crucial.

Because of the utmost importance accorded to breastfeeding in the parenting relationship, attachment mothers seldom shared the job of infant feeding with anyone (fathers or otherwise). There was a strong sense that the mother was irreplaceable. Indeed, amongst these mothers a certain amount of anger was directed towards those who 'clamour for involvement' (Amelia), by trying to 'help' feed the baby – again, particularly in the early months, when it was understood as important that the mother and child 'bond'. Arguably, if a woman invests a lot of identity work in her ability to breastfeed her child, attempts by others to feed the baby will be seen as a threat to that very status.

Feminism?

The attachment mothers I spoke with refer to themselves as feminists, using a cultural framework that accommodates and celebrates essential differences between women and men. They consider themselves informed consumers who have 'chosen' traditional set-ups (and it is this *choice* that separates them from the stereotypical 1950s housewife [Bobel 2002]). At the same time – for Jan, at least – the family set-up is a reflection of a natural state of being:

Questionnaire: What does it mean to be a parent?

Jan [32, breastfeeding her 8-month-old daughter]: Being there for your child, being loving, filling the child's needs, guiding the child, encouraging his development.

Questionnaire: What does it mean to be a mother?

Jan: Obviously the same but I think the mother has a more intense role especially if she is breastfeeding. Nature intended mothers to be responsible for nourishing their babies and so with this responsibility another level develops in the relationship. My family is classic: mother, father, child and I am happy about this. There are lots of other types of families now and I am sure they create loving relationships. I can't say if one is better than the other because I only know my experience.

Questionnaire: Is there a difference between these two questions?

Jan: I think the mother has a special role and a special relationship with the child. If the mother is not there I don't know what effect that has on the child, I'm sure it depends on many variables. I am just happy to be a mother and hope I will be able to be there for [my child] for a long time.

As Bobel notes, feeding norms, which are so central to this form of parenting, over time 'established caring patterns that persisted throughout mothers' and fathers' parenting careers' (Bobel 2002: 134). So when women talked about their childcare practices in later life – such as when the child had reached the age of three or four – this biological narrative remained the most important rationalisation for the mother's full time-caring, despite the fact that the breastfeeding by this point had generally dwindled to a few times a day:

Signe [Leader applicant, 30, breastfeeding her 3-year-old son]: I just know what he wants, you know? And I can provide it. When I put him to bed it takes about two minutes with a quick breastfeed; if [husband] tries to do it, it can take him two hours.

Patricia's comment also highlights how biological narratives intersect with structural realities, which means she spends all her time with the baby and is the one with the time to read up about attachment parenting methods. This in turn, has had repercussions far beyond getting the baby fed:

Patricia [30, breastfeeding her 1-year-old son. Questionnaire response, emphasis added]: The only downside I feel is that I have to do this on my own and although [my husband] is very supportive I am aware that part of him would like me to breastfeed less so that his involvement could be more, and [my son's] dependence on me would lessen. I also feel that [my husband] has no support or source of information (or time to read), so that everything he learns comes from me (from LLL groups and reading etc) so that, for example, he was quite shocked when I said I would probably be breastfeeding for a few more years. He said he felt left out of the decision-making on that. Also breastfeeding is tied to almost everything else you do as a mother, most of all how you comfort your child and how you get them to sleep. *So I feel quite responsible for being the driving force behind key decisions that we make about how we parent.*

Intensive Fathering?

A notable development in UK policy has been an 'intensification' of fathering, with calls for fathers to be more 'involved' in the care of their children with the aim of 'mending' the fabric of society (see, e.g., Jack Straw's 'Lads need Dads' arguments made in 2007, BBC 2007). It is interesting to explore the contradiction between styles of parenting that argue for mother-child attachment on the one hand, and calls for gender equality and paternal engagement on the other. Dr Sears, the attachment parenting author, notes that although fathers might not have this 'irrefutable biology', they nevertheless have 'natural nurturing abilities' that should be developed: 'Although mothers do indeed have a hormonal head start on developing their intuition, I believe that fathers also have natural nurturing abilities, and, if given the opportunity to develop these abilities, fathers can indeed participate in the care and comforting of their babies' (Sears 2003).

Yet despite this discourse, mothers almost always remain full-time, primary caregivers to their children (Wall and Arnold 2007). Indeed, despite an emphasis on the 'modern' style of fathering, some ambiguity lingers about what 'intensive' or 'involved' fathering really means in practice, apart from assertions of what it is not (i.e., 'uninvolved' and unlike one's own father) (Dermott 2008). In general, in her study of fathers, Dermott (2008) found that whereas notions of emotional openness, communication and a close relationship with one's children were endorsed, a wide variety of childcare and labour patterns were possible under the hazy 'involved' fathering rubric.

Certainly, the 'irrefutable biology' of mothering became a source of tension for some couples. Lauren, who recounted her 'typical day' in Chapter 3, told this story about her relationship later in the same interview:

> *Lauren [42, breastfeeding her 2½-year-old daughter, emphasis added]*: And having a child is wonderful … but my couple is such a mess, it is in tatters.
>
> *Charlotte*: Really?
>
> *Lauren*: I think that maybe you don't know a man until you have a child with him. The jealousy that my husband would feel when I was breastfeeding was unbelievable. For me, it's your child, and breast-feeding is the best thing you can do for them but then you have this stupid arsed husband who would say 'ah! you've been breastfeed-ing all day long haven't you?' And I've heard that quite a lot of men are jealous, and I find that quite pathetic. But because I am quite headstrong…. ([To her child]: Booby? No? Bye bye booby?) I have a strong relationship with my daughter, we are very close, physically. But with my husband, it is a catastrophe. And we are doing counsel-ling, but I don't know, I think it is useless to be honest.
>
> *Charlotte*: I'm sorry.
>
> *Lauren*: Well, he has moved here on the sofa bed … she is getting big-ger and takes more space. So he moved here. And erm, we just sleep so badly the three together in the same bed. If he were in harmony with us it would be possible, but he doesn't understand the harmony. I mean when she turns, I turn. I mean, that's a bit of a cliché, but there is something in it. A man and a woman sleep together in a cer-tain way, and a man and a baby and woman sleep together in a dif-ferent way. *And my husband just doesn't fit into this threesome at all.* And he was sleeping so badly. So he migrated onto the sofa bed, which actually suits me so well, you know. Maybe it's the road to divorce. I don't know, I don't care. I'm fed up…. *My baby is my priority. And I have always said it. And I have spoken to my other women friends and they say of course your baby is your priority! It is biological.* And I just think that it is maybe something men just can't understand, and get jealous about or something. And I don't know, maybe it triggers feelings of abandon-ment or something. Who knows?
>
> But my priority is definitely with my child. Of course I would love to split up from my husband, but I am financially dependent on him. And I think the world is in the state that it is now because women are busy raising their children, and the world is left to these stupid men who are immature, big children.

Although this case was rare, it was certainly true that attachment mothers often felt a need to balance their intimacy with their child (or children) and their partner, who might otherwise feel excluded.

To this end, women would frequently talk about being 'touched-out' by breastfeeding their children and thus disinclined to be in physical contact with their partners, again highlighting the physicality of this style of mothering. Some women worried about their partners being jealous, but the majority seemed to think this was immature on the part of the husband, who should be more supportive. In line with an intensive mothering framework, the child's needs come first:

> *Charlotte*: And when you say it's pleasurable [breastfeeding], do you worry about saying that?
>
> *Leticia [36, 3½-year-old son, breastfeeding her 2-year-old daughter]*: No.… There is always the element where you are getting intimacy satisfaction from your child, but your partner is missing out … there is an imbalance, and the partner can feel quite … jealous or feel quite left out. Left out I guess is the big aspect … the partner has to make peace with that, it is a temporary thing, and that for the next year or year and a half the mother is going to have that physical connection with the baby. And to some extent the mother can compensate for that by going out of her way to be physical with the partner, when perhaps she doesn't have the impulse.

Exploring the challenges families face in maintaining their philosophical choices opens up the relationship between choice and accountability. Gayle points to some of these tensions in her response, which is highly gendered:

> *Questionnaire*: Is there a difference between these two [definitions of mother and parent]?
>
> *Gayle [32, breastfeeding her 8-month-old daughter. Questionnaire response, emphasis added]*: I do think there is a difference between mothers and fathers; but as I am a mother and a parent the question is the same. I think that fathers find it easier to sustain their sense of self. *I feel as if my whole self is subordinated to her, and that that is how it should be.* I think my partner feels the same way, but I also think he has a more innate sense that he should also have a 'self' outside of this. But whether this is character or gender it is not possible to say.

Cultural Contradictions of Going Natural

Even though full-term breastfeeding and attachment parenting might be 'natural', they require considerable diligence, attentiveness and effort on the part of mothers (arguably as much as methods at the more 'structured' end of the childcare spectrum, despite the more liberal discourse). The strain of this effort was evident at LLL groups, where women occasionally arrived at a meeting and promptly burst into tears. They would talk about how they were utterly shattered from not sleeping properly over a period of years (particularly the case if they continued to share a bed with their child, as was typical). One woman told me she had not slept for a period of more than four hours in the five years since her daughter's birth. This might also be the case with some parents who do not co-sleep or breastfeed to 'full term', but it is important to recognise the embodied maternal labour inherent to this approach.

The Searses, who gave attachment *parenting* its name, now include a seventh 'tool' in their list – Balance – after seeing too many cases of what they call 'mother burnout' (Sears and Sears 2001: 112) and not, interestingly, 'parent burnout'. Women at the meetings met with much sympathy from other mothers and shared stories of broken sleep. 'You are doing a wonderful job,' they were usually told. Yet the counsel was generally to persevere. They were reassured that it was normal to feel this way, and that in time it would pass.

The articulation of 'natural truths' that stress mothers' availability to children often contrasts to the actual experiences, and indeed, identities, of many mothers today (Buskens 2001). Following Hays (1996), it is suggested here that in the social and economic context of post-industrialised societies, following perceived natural patterns of lactation creates a 'cultural contradiction' for the women doing it.

Numerous anthropologists and historians have shown how intensive caregiving carried out by biological mothers in the private sphere is a result of modern economic and political arrangements (Ariès 1962; Badinter 1981; Blaffer Hrdy 2000; Engels 1972; Maher 1992). Yet proponents of 'natural' or 'attachment' parenting seem 'blissfully unaware' (to quote Buskens 2001: 79) of the social differences between a hunter-gatherer society and those of mothers in contemporary Britain. Buskens (2001) shows how mothering as a post-enlightenment practice has intensified through the emphasis on 'good mothering', but this has taken place in a context of diminishing support with the loss of coherent community. The approach eclipses the social surroundings of women – and the presence or otherwise of 'alloparents', who share the job of parenting. Blaffer Hrdy (2000), for example, points out that where possible, mothers 'in African societies' may seek to extend infant and child care to helpers (including fathers) to improve their own productivity. Yet a gendered split in British society has rendered motherhood an isolated business for mothers. 'Mothers are thus attempting to carry out rigorous schedules of attached mothering in an increasingly fragmented and unsupportive social context,' says Buskens (2001: 81). (It will be interesting to see how, if at all, the new parental leave measures noted in Chapter 2 might influence this.)

Early childhood *is* a period of high emotional and physical dependency. This is not just an invention of an intensive parenting culture. As Buskens argues, 'infants do require a long period of intensive, embodied nurture. *The problem is not the fact of this requirement but rather that meeting this need has come to rest exclusively, and in isolation, on the shoulders of biological mothers.* This historically novel situation is precisely what is left unsaid and therefore unproblematized in popular accounts of "natural" parenting' (Buskens 2001: 81, emphasis in original).

To expect 'natural' styles of parenting in a society that lacks traditional structures is to force a 'cultural contradiction' on women, since one cannot, argues Buskens, live comfortably outside the dominant values of their social structure. It therefore has profound implications on women's identity work:

> Following the prescribed parenting practice creates for mothers an ontological and physical condition that cannot readily be accommodated in the structures of modern society. The result is either social exclusion or the exhaustion of trying to combine normative opposites (home and work, public and private, childcare and leisure). This is a contradiction at the heart of modern culture that cannot be ameliorated by spurious returns to nature or by appeals to an already invented tradition. (Buskens 2001: 84)

To reiterate, management of this contradiction is affected by socioeconomic status. That almost all women interviewed were with a partner, white and well-educated, and that over half were not working outside the home, tells us yet again that more is at stake here than a simple exercise of choice.

A Return to Anthropology?

In her talk 'Tracing the Mirage of Space between Nature and Nurture,'[10] Fox Keller reflected on the current fascination with distinguishing cultural from natural influences on human development. Despite work that has effectively silenced the debate (by showing that the environment influences expression of genetic phenotype), she noted that we continue to separate the two. Marilyn Strathern, listening to the talk, agreed. 'I thought I had answered this question back in 1982', she said, 'but the same ideas keep getting recycled.' Why do 'nature' and 'culture' retain such explanatory power? Earlier, Strathern had traced the nature/culture distinction back to Levi-Strauss (and beyond) to argue that

> Nature and culture tend to acquire certain meanings as categories of analysis when those working mainly in an empiricist tradition turn to the exegesis of cognitive systems ... nature and culture are understood in an essentialist sense: that is, peoples apparently entertaining notions of this order may be thought of as wrestling with the same problems of control and definition as form the content of these terms for ourselves. (Strathern 1982: 177)

This is, notes Strathern, not least because the social sciences tend to employ certain constituents of the nature/culture matrix, including those concerned with ecological systems and their environments, and society and the 'individual' (Strathern 1982: 177). She comments that a long tradition in European thought has concerned the opposition between things as they are and things as they might be: separation of the subject from object as part of a dialectic between participation and objectivity: 'The combined capacity to participate in "otherness" and treat that otherness as an object (of study) has made anthropology' (Strathern 1982: 177). But crucially, this depends upon the assumption that humans 'make' culture in so far as we can stand outside of our own 'nature'.

The anthropological discipline itself is to blame for notions of the primitive (and the primate) as conduits for understanding an essential humanity, since their utility in this task depends on a separation of 'culture' from a baseline 'nature', a division that has been foundational to the discipline as a science. In my own accounts of social life, utilising the same categories my informants used has complicated an anthropological analysis of evolutionary discourses for the naturality of breastfeeding – particularly as the categories are so fundamental to the anthropological discipline itself.

Yet the production of knowledge is, for Haraway (1978b), collective storytelling. In repeating the approach of the past (by searching for origins), feminists 'have allowed the theory of the body politic to be split in such a way that natural knowledge is being reincorporated covertly into techniques of social control instead of being transformed into sciences of liberation' (Haraway 1978: 23). A feminist history of science, however, 'could examine that part of biosocial science in which our alleged evolutionary biology is traced and supposedly inevitable patterns of order based on domination are legitimated. The examination should play seriously with the rich ambiguity and metaphorical possibilities of both technical and ordinary words ... to discover and to define what is "natural" for ourselves' (Haraway 1978b: 39). Haraway does not dismiss primatology, then, but rather says that we must *use* the biosocial sciences from 'the point of view of the process of resolving the contradiction between, or the gap between, human reality and human possibility in history' (Haraway 1978b: 60). Blaffer Hrdy is one author she cites as engaging in this task.

Blaffer Hrdy's book *Mother Nature* (2000) aims to use sociobiological thinking to show how mothers throughout the animal world, especially amongst primates and throughout hominid development, make conscious and unconscious decisions about their investment in offspring based on ecological circumstances, maternal condition, the existence and age of prior offspring, and perceived infant viability (Hausman 2003: 150). Maternal decisions are not arbitrary, then, but have always been about weighing up the odds. Blaffer Hrdy writes that as birth intervals grew shorter through the course of human evolution and recent human history, pressure on mothers to delegate caretaking to others became more intense. Whenever they safely could, or when they had little choice, mothers handed babies over to fathers or alloparents, weaned them early, or swaddled them and hung them from doors. At the psychological level, these decisions differ little from those a contemporary mother makes every day when she asks her neighbour to babysit or contracts for more or less adequate day care. She is playing the odds and evaluating her priorities (Blaffer Hrdy 2000: 379).

The historical response, when newborns seem less likely to survive, when their survival might endanger that of an older sibling, or when the mother feels investing in the infant would be dangerous to her own survival, has been infanticide or abandonment (Blaffer Hrdy [2000: 288–317], discussed in Hausman [2003: 151]; Maher's [1992] collection makes a similar point). As Hausman notes, Blaffer Hrdy's chapter on 'Unnatural Mothers' shows how those mothers most likely to be perceived as unnatural were in fact only responding appropriately to difficult situations: in adverse circumstances it was the females who carried babies to term who were 'unnatural', not those who did not. Blaffer Hrdy successfully includes mothers as agents within the evolutionary framework by avoiding a narrow focus on the infants around whom maternal behaviour is held to adapt. Blaffer Hrdy argues that mothers are constantly making decisions on a cost-benefit analysis. As Hausman says:

> Feeding with formula, especially when mothers know (as most American mothers do) that breast milk is better for their infants, is one way of reducing the cost to one's own body, and in some ways (Hrdy might also argue) of reducing one's investment in offspring. Reducing maternal investment in offspring, if even by a little bit, can provide a breathing space for mothers expected to be sacrificial, attentive, and ever-patient. (Hausman 2003: 151)

Thus, 'humans manipulate infant feeding because we can' (Hausman 2003: 152). To suggest that breastfeeding is biologically beneficial to babies and that this fact should determine women's actions is to leave aside other constraints in women's lives that determine what Blaffer Hrdy refers to as 'the Hamilton Equation' – defining altruistic behaviour in relation to cost to giver and genetic relatedness. As Hausman writes: 'Humans have discovered how to manipulate infant feeding (although the jury is still out on some of the biological and social effects of not nursing at all) through thousands, perhaps hundreds of thousands of years of trial and error with a variety of substances and care arrangements' (Hausman 2003: 152). The quote from the LLL book at the start of this section states: 'Human beings' ideas about when and how to wean are often determined by culture, not necessarily by what is best or natural for babies and mothers.' This narrow view of what is 'best' validates a heavily gendered notion of appropriate care. Women nevertheless appropriate the rationale in the course of their identity work, as it puts their role as primary carers beyond debate: it is what nature intended.

Haraway does not discount primatological, or even cross-cultural, cross-temporal research in attempts to understand humanity; in fact, she is 'edified' by it. '*Primate Visions* does not work by prohibiting origin stories, or biological explanations of what some would insist must be exclusively cultural matters … I am not interested in policing the boundaries between nature and culture – quite opposite, I am edified by the traffic,' she writes (Haraway 1989: 377). 'Re-map[ping] the borderlands between nature and culture' is her invitation. I do so here by looking at a 'culture of being natural' in parenting. Analysis of the rhetorical effects of evolutionary narratives in the creation of this culture clearly has repercussions beyond parenting.

Postscript

In an interview, two mothers discuss another mother:

> *Rachel [41, breastfeeding her 3-year-old son]*: I have a friend who has a
> son at the same age of [my son] and managed to breastfeed for about
> a year then stopped ... and she was really into natural childbirth and
> that sort of thing ... and we saw them the other day, and we were
> talking about extended breastfeeding, and she was saying 'it's all very
> well that it's natural but you have to take into consideration how so-
> ciety is'. You know, 'it might be natural, but that doesn't mean you
> have to do it'. I was surprised that was her attitude.

> *Lila [37, breastfeeding her 4-year-old son]*: ... people are so out of touch,
> you know?

> *Rachel*: Yeah, it might be that it's what society says, but that doesn't
> mean it is right or good! It gives me more reason *not* to do what soci-
> ety says, but, you know.

> *Lila*: Society is just so detached now. Nobody is in touch with any-
> thing. The same with the environment. Just because everyone is driv-
> ing a car doesn't make it right, you know. People don't have a clue
> what food looks like. We are just all about ready-made meals. There
> are so many people who don't know what real vegetables look like. It
> makes formula feeding more natural. That's the tragedy of our time.

Notes

1. In the quote from Megan, there is slippage between 'normal' and 'natural'. What this respondent is doing – breastfeeding her 4-year-old son
   – is not 'normal' in the statistical sense, but she uses the authority of
   the word to justify what she does as normal in terms of the expression
   of 'natural' physiological processes. See Chapter 5.
2. Ball has found that breastfed infants who sleep in their mother's bed
   have their needs (for warmth, food and comfort) attended to more
   rapidly, and that their mothers to get more rest than those who put
   their babies in separate cots. Because of concerns about the safety of
   having infants in the same bed, the NHS is now considering whether
   to attach 'side-cots' to maternity beds rather than using separate stand-
   alone cots (Ball 2007).
3. This section draws on Small's chapter 'Food for Thought' (1998: 177–
   212). Information shared at LLL meetings is also used in the discussion
   here.
4. Linnaeus, writing in 1758, devised the term *mammalia,* or 'of the
   breast', to determine a class of animals that lactate. For Schiebinger,

in 'so doing, he idolized the female mammae as the icon of that class' (1993: 40). Indeed, it was not a common-sense term, as it refers only to a subset of half of a group of animals (females), namely, those that lactate (for a short period of time, or not at all):

> By honouring the mammae as a sign and symbol of the highest class of animals, Linnaeus assigned a new value to the female, especially women's unique role in reproduction ... yet in the same edition, also introduced homo sapiens (man of wisdom) to distinguish humans from other primates. ...Thus, with Linnaean terminology, a female characteristic (the lactating mammae) ties humans to brutes, while a traditionally male characteristic (reason) marks out separateness. (Schiebinger 1993: 53–55).

5. It is interesting to note that recent research into the age of weaning in prehistoric communities actually tends to put it at between 2 and 4 years old, as opposed to 6 or 7 (Clayton, Sealy and Pfeiffer 2006).

6. For the most part, women did not see any contradiction in being 'natural'. The only woman I met during the course of fieldwork who seemed aware of any tensions had conceived her child with the aid of IVF techniques. 'If it were all left to nature', Vicky said, looking at her daughter, 'we wouldn't even be here, would we?' Indeed, she points to an interesting area of debate within anthropology itself. Strathern (1992a, 1992b) notes that nature has increasingly become so 'assisted' by technology that it can no longer provide prior ontological status to culture; at the same time, 'nature' clearly provides some sort of model for 'culture' here.

7. For McCaughey (2008), author of *The Caveman Mystique*, evolutionary narratives applied to women are highly prescriptive. Those applied to men, however – the cavemen who 'naturally' want to impregnate many women – they are descriptive. Given my informants' endorsement of full-term breastfeeding with a physiological rubric, their answers to the question of the 'naturality' of marriage (or monogamy) were confusing. Veronika uses the 'primitive' to mirror her monogamous relationship:

> *Charlotte*: But is marriage natural? Physiologically men would be impregnating...
>
> *Veronika*: Not in all cultures, do men do that.

8. Some informants resented the use of the word 'father' in the LLL philosophy, preferring 'mother's partner' instead.

9. Breastfeeding is frequently said to be the one thing that men can't do for children. In fact, there have been cases reported of men lactating – producing a colostrum-like substance in extreme or unusual circumstances (Menstuff 2011). Whether this can be done 'at will' is another matter. Despite many women telling me of this capacity of the male breast, I never heard of any couples actually using this technique to share the job of feeding/comforting their children.

10. Centre for Research in the Arts Social Sciences and Humanities, Cambridge, 22 March 2007.

Chapter 7

'WHAT SCIENCE SAYS IS BEST'
SCIENCE AS DOGMA

When women told me that what they were doing was 'most natural', they did not mean they were blindly following the examples of 'primitives' or primates. They also *knew* that what they were doing was best for their children because 'science' tells them it is healthiest. Science 'reveals' nature (Jordanova 1986: 29). There is an informed reflexivity to the predetermined 'natural' pattern that women follow.

Attachment mothers use the term 'science' to refer to evidence derived from physiological and psychological studies concerning developmental and health benefits of full-term breastfeeding and attachment parenting. The intention here is to unpack the saliency of their assertions within the intensive motherhood framework. 'Health', a primary rationale women use in making decisions about how to feed their infants, sits well in a paradigm of liberal democracy where citizens are urged to 'Choose Health' (see Chapter 2). Women's use of the discourses of science is a critical element of their identity work, serving as an accountability strategy par excellence, which – like recourse to nature – serves to edify their marginal position and foreclose further debate about their non-conventional breastfeeding.

'Science' is not a discourse confined to parenting, of course – it is probably *the* dominant culture in post-industrial societies. Erikson (2005) remarks:

> We live with science: science surrounds us, invades our lives, and alters our perspective on the world. We see things from a scientific

perspective, in that we use science to help us make sense of the world – regardless of whether or not that is an appropriate thing to do – and to legitimise the picture of the world that results from such investigations. (Erikson 2005: 224, in McCaughey 2008: 9)

As noted, it is ironic that the women here use science as one of their accountability strategies, since many attachment parenting advocates are openly sceptical about scientific knowledge. Some attachment parents refuse to vaccinate their children owing to belief in a causal link (between the MMR vaccine and autism, in the most famous case) or the presence of dangerously high levels of toxins in vaccines (Robinson 2007; see Fitzpatrick [2004] for an account of the MMR debates). My interest here is in the selective use (and misuse) of scientific evidence to support certain (moral) discourses about parenting.

Throughout this chapter, 'science' is understood as a 'situated knowledge' (Haraway 1988). This conception is a means of calling to attention the fact that science has bearing on reality 'out there' at the same time that its truth claims, and their application to parenting practices, require contextualisation. As Latour's work made evident, science does not merely represent 'nature' (itself a representation) but embodies the interests of the social actors involved in its production (Latour 1993). To some extent, this chapter explores the relationship between science and society, whilst acknowledging that the production of scientific knowledge is a deeply social project. Corsín Jiménez notes a transformation in the means of producing scientific knowledge, in that the validation of knowledge as scientifically robust is no longer a project for scientists alone: 'Today, society decides what makes good science' (Jiménez 2007: 39).

The Scientific Claim for Full-Term Breastfeeding and Attachment Parenting

As Sinnott (2010) notes, the limited number of studies concerning long-term breastfeeding have largely been conducted in the developing world, which complicates comparison with the UK context (Persson et al. 1998; Taren and Chen, 1993). One of the few studies in the US noted little more than that in thirty-eight children breastfed between 12 and 43 months, growth patterns were in 'normal' ranges (Buckley, 2001). The website www.kellymom.com, which many of my informants referred to frequently, has an 'extended breastfeeding factsheet' in which Kelly Bonyata, a lactation consultant (IBCLC) from the US, collates much of the research on breastfeeding in toddlerhood. The fact sheet focuses on nutritional benefits, showing how breast milk continues to be a source of nutrients, including vitamins and folates, at whatever age it is consumed (Dewey 2001). Indeed, because breastfeeding works on a supply-demand basis, breast milk consumed by a child nursing less often will be more concentrated in these nutrients and immunological substances (Goldman, Garsa and Goldblum 1983).

The available research shows that nursing toddlers are ill less often than their formula-fed peers (Gulick 1986), although it is probable that those children who are breastfed into toddlerhood are also less likely to be surrounded by other children in childcare centres and other facilities (there may also be a reporting bias on the part of parents here). Bonyata says that 'extensive research' on the relationship between IQ and length of breastfeeding has shown a correlative increase, though the fact sheet (which in any event should be read cautiously) does not refer to any studies supporting this claim. Bonyata cites Kniedel (1990), who, writing in *New Beginnings*, a periodical for LLLI leaders, claims there is no evidence that continued breastfeeding interferes with a child's ability or desire to eat other foods. Mothers themselves are also said to benefit from continuing to breastfeed, as the risk of developing a range of cancers decreases in correlation with time spent breastfeeding; however, the strength of this evidence is questionable.

But the scientific claim for extended breastfeeding goes beyond actual feeding in terms of the transmission of breast milk from mother to child. More often, arguments are made about the 'whole approach to parenting' that typically coalesces around this practice – attachment parenting.

Beyond evolutionary studies, the 'science' on attachment parenting is limited – if only because a limited amount of research has been conducted, on a limited number of children. Evidence in favour of attachment parenting comes from two major bodies of work: psychological studies with a focus on attachment anxieties (stemming from the work of Bowlby, Ainsworth and others in the 1950s), and neuroscience-informed work drawing on studies of brain development (e.g., Gerhardt 2004, Sunderland 2006). It is worth reiterating here that there is no evidence that full-term breastfeeding is harmful, either psychologically or physiologically, but nor is there evidence that parenting in 'normal' (i.e., non-attachment ways) is damaging. What follows is a contextualisation of the claims that attachment parenting is positively beneficial.

Psychological Evidence

The work of Bowlby and Ainsworth in the 1950s and 1960s forms the basis of what is now known as attachment theory (Ainsworth et al. 1962, Bowlby 1969; see also discussion in Chapter 2). Following observation of mother-infant pairs, the mother came to be understood as the infant's base of 'secure attachment'. The term refers to an infant's behaviour during the 'strange situation' test Ainsworth devised for children over a year old: a child is left alone in a room with a stranger, and the child's behaviour on seeing the parent again is the basis for classification into levels of attachment. The clinical definition of a securely attached infant is one who is distressed when the parent leaves, but easily comforted on their return. Bowlby (1969, 2005) argued that if the mother was absent (either physically or mentally) during the formative period of attachment, the child could suffer disorders such as anxiety or depression. This finding was rooted in the belief that the mother-child bond is the linchpin of infant development, determining a child's ability to cope with future relationships (see Kanieski 2010).

Yet the evidence in support of this theory of 'attachment' has been called into question. Eyer notes that rather than being tied to a consistent primary attachment figure, or restricted to a specific sensitive period, 'attachment' should be considered a highly plastic phenomenon amongst human beings (Eyer 1992: 69). It is also important to note a nominative slippage here: attachment parenting, as a specific way of raising children, has little correlation with Bowlby's attachment theory: practices such as co-sleeping, breastfeeding and baby wearing are not necessarily tied to the development of greater attachment in mother-infant pairs.

The secure attachment or 'strange situation' test is also problematic as a defence of attachment parenting methods. According to a meta-analysis of studies using the test (van Ijzendoorn and Kroonberg 1988), 75 per cent of British babies tested in 1988 were securely attached – at a time when bottle-feeding and separate sleeping occurred at even higher rates in Britain than today. In the 'primitive societies' that attachment parenting advocates consider to exhibit ideal parenting – such as the Gusili mothers of Kenya, who wear their babies, breastfeed into toddlerhood and respond quickly to their babies' crying – only 61 per cent of babies were shown to be securely attached. This might, of course, say something about the cross-cultural applicability of such a test – in that case, though, there is no way of comparing psychological well-being cross-culturally, and little argument that replicating 'primitive' parenting in contemporary Britain is superior to other forms of care. If the test is applicable cross-culturally, then there is clearly little correlation between attachment parenting and the rate of securely attached babies.[1]

Furthermore, even though some research has shown that mothers who are sensitive and responsive to their infants' needs are more likely to have 'securely attached' children, the mother-infant dyads studied have not included mothers who show atypically high levels of involvement with their children. Empirical research on maternal overprotectiveness shows an association with raised levels of anxiety in children, suggesting that high-intensity attachment parenting could actually lead to insecure rather than secure attachment relationships between children and their mothers (McNamara 2006; however, there is little research on this topic).

Yet Bowlby and Ainsworth's ideas remain influential in mainstream parenting discourses, as well as amongst women breastfeeding long-term. LLL states that the mother-baby relationship 'sets the prototype for other relationships throughout life' (LLL 2004: 185). Many women in my sample referred to Bowlby's work when explaining their decision to carry out full-term breastfeeding and attachment parenting. Child-centred care, with mothers responding quickly to their infants' 'cues', was said to be a primary means of bringing about secure attachment. For example, Sally, quoted in Chapter 3, says she hopes her daughter will be quite a 'secure person' in her teenage years after having had her 'fill of being held and touched and breastfed'.

In this vein Veronika Robinson writes, in defence of full-term breastfeeding: 'It has been shown that long-term breastfeeding children were more able to form attachments to others, and to become more independent than their bottle-fed peers. In adolescence, these teenagers considered that their mothers weren't over-protective, but more caring' (Robinson 2007: 154). She makes this claim with reference to the following literature:

Ainsworth M. 1973. 'The development of infant-mother attachment.' In Caldwell. BM. Ricciuiti, HN. (Eds.) *Review of Child Development Research*. University of Chicago Press, Chicago.

Fergussen DM. Woodward LJ. 1999. 'Breastfeeding and later psycho-social adjustment.' *Pediatri Perinatol Epidemiol* 13: 114–157.

In using the phrase 'it has been shown', Robinson presents the work of Ainsworth and Fergussen and Woodward as definitive evidence of the benefits of full-term breastfeeding, though in fact, neither of these authors' work gives such evidence about attachment levels in long-term breastfeeding children per se.

Robinson's book *The Drinks Are On Me* (2007) was written after her appearance on the *Extraordinary Breastfeeding* documentary, for which she received a lot of publicity. Her book is written as a response to her critics and, like many of the attachment mothers here, she uses the language of science to defend and validate her choices. For example, she writes:

When women once again listen to their intuitive voice, they'll know that although raising a child naturally takes an enormous amount of time and energy, it also brings a beautiful and irreplaceable, intimate connection. The children of such women won't form attachments to inanimate objects [such as dummies or comfort blankets] in the hopes of getting their needs met. *Instead, they'll form healthy, life-long relationships, and most importantly, will not be afraid to love* (53). Studies reveal a much lower divorce rate amongst people who received long-term breastfeeding as children (61). (Robinson 2007: 145; emphasis in original)

The references from the last two sentences are:

53: See the work of Pam Chubbuck for further information. Breastfeeding is essential for bio-psycho-spiritual health, Pam Chubbuck, PhD.

61: Breastfeeding: brain nutrients in brain development for human love and peace. See table 1, James Prescotts's *www.violence.de/prescott.ttf/article.html*[2]

Pam Chubbuck's website describes her as a 'pastoral counsellor', a psychotherapist and member of the International Faculty of the Institute of Core Energetics. She is also an LLL leader. Prescott's work draws upon Textor's *A Cross Cultural Summary* (1967), offering evidence from twenty societies where the weaning age is over 2½ years of age to argue that these societies have lower divorce rates than those where the weaning age is earlier. It is somewhat problematic to compare rates of divorce in pre- and post-industrialised societies, if one accepts that marriage is as much an economic arrangement as an expression of love through kinship bonds. Yet combining this with other evolutionary arguments, Prescott states:

> In summary, the lessons to be learned are clear. If *Homo Sapiens* is to survive as a species, he/she must return to the 'life plan' of Mother Gaia who, through her wisdom of millions of years of evolutionary biology and socio-biology, has provided for the intimate physical affectional bonding between mother and her offspring which establishes the foundation for later sensual affectional bonding and for human love itself. For without human love there can be no survival of *Homo Sapiens*. (Prescott, 1997)

Claims that 'studies reveal a much lower divorce rate amongst people who received long-term breastfeeding as children' – implying that this has been shown through randomised controlled trials – lend themselves the appearance of scientific authority. This trope is common in arguments made by attachment parenting advocates, who often use such phrases as 'science says' or 'studies have shown' to legitimate moral arguments about the importance of particular styles of care. A further example is given by the Searses, whose book states, 'Science says: AP Infants thrive' (Sears and Sears 2001: 18). Throughout their book, the Searses present similar 'Science says' boxes, glossing a slippage between animals and humans through the language of science: 'Experiments on both human infants and infant experimental animals showed these fascinating results: (1) Human infants with the most secure attachment to their mothers had the best cortisol balance. (2) The longer infant animals were separated from their mothers, the higher their cortisol levels, suggesting these babies [animals] could be chronically stressed' (Sears and Sears 2001: 18).

There is a gap, then, between (real) 'science' and the way in which 'science' is mobilised. As Wolfenstein noted back in 1955:

> [E]xperts draw upon a growing body of knowledge about children. But the process of transmission of scientific findings in this field is not simple or direct. Findings remain incomplete and their implications for practice often ambiguous. Those who mediate between science and the lay public often draw on their own and currently prevailing moral attitudes to derive practical recommendations. Thus child-training literature is as much expressive of the moral climate of the time and place in which it is written as of the state of scientific knowledge about children. (Wolfenstein 1955: 145)

Neuroscience: 'Real Evidence'

Increasingly, attachment parenting advocates refer to neuroscientific work to strengthen their claims. This is a 'breakthrough', as an article in *Mothering Magazine* (to which I was referred by the LLL member in the US cited in the introduction) puts it, since proponents of attachment theory have, until recently, had little 'unbiased and testable information' with which to back up their claims:

> In our society, attachment parenting is seen as just another of an array of parenting options, and is typically viewed as the most difficult and least appealing choice. What is missing is the science that modern assessment methods and technology can offer. Now, with the ability to study the intricacies of the brain and its functioning on a cellular level, science can deliver conclusive data to back up each aspect of Bowlby's comprehensive theory, and then some. The data are powerful and offer what no other parenting model puts forward: unbiased and testable information about the workings of the infant brain and the effects of both stress and health on brain development. (Porter 2003)

In the UK, writers such as Gerhardt (*Why Love Matters: How Affection Shapes a Baby's Brain,* 2004) and Sunderland (*The Science of Parenting,* 2006) have drawn on neuroscientific work looking at the interactions between parents and children and how these affect the structure of the infant brain. The argument is that from late pregnancy through into the second year of life, the human brain undergoes a critical period of accelerated growth. With the use of MRI scans and other technologies, interaction between the development of the brain and the social environment (nature and nurture) can (arguably) be observed. As the *Mothering Magazine* article states: 'What has emerged is mounting evidence that stress and trauma impair optimal brain development while healthy attachment promotes it.'[3] The article continues: 'Babies, we know, cannot survive on their own. All basic needs must be met through a relationship with a caregiver. ... In order to maintain emotional equilibrium, babies require a consistent and committed relationship with one caring person. As you might expect, the research indicates that the person best suited for this relationship is the mother.'[4]

The Womanly Art of Breastfeeding makes a similar point:

> So it is not surprising that a recent study found that more human contact makes for a happier baby. Those babies who spent more time

being held or carried either in mother's arms or in a baby carrier – even while contented or asleep – cried less. The younger the baby, the more dramatic were the results. Three extra hours of carrying a day reduced the amount of crying in a four-week-old infant by forty-five percent. (LLLI 2004: 78)

The claim made is that during the early stages of distress – perhaps at the absence of the mother, as in the strange situation test – a baby's heart rate, blood pressure and respiration are heightened, to which the brain responds by releasing stress hormones, elevating the brain's levels of adrenalin, noradrenaline and dopamine (Brown 1982). Should the distress continue, the infant may go into 'shutdown mode' – a survival strategy allowing the infant to restore homeostasis. Prolonged periods in this state have damaging effects on the development of the infant brain. Because the infant is in distress, the 'regulatory resources' of the body are all dedicated to maintaining equilibrium, rather than focused on 'normal' growth and development:

'These kind of biochemical alterations in the rapidly developing right brain have long-lasting effects. In the infant, states become traits, so the effects of such early relational traumas become part of the structure of the forming personality.'[5] The focus on restoring equilibrium can, according to this argument, permanently alter the chemistry of the brain to the extent that 'states becomes traits', and the child's personality is shaped accordingly; children who experience stress in early life, it is argued, are more susceptible to mental health disorders in later life.

Following this argument, when parents respond to their baby's cues (of happiness, distress or otherwise) they can be said to be ensuring optimal development. As Gerhardt (2004) puts it:

When parents respond to the baby's signals, they are participating in many important biological processes. They are helping the baby's nervous system to mature in such a way that it does not get overstressed. They are helping the bioamine pathways to be set at a moderate level. They are helping to build up the prefrontal cortex and the child's capacity to hold information in mind, to reflect on feeling, to restrain impulses, that will be a vital part of his or her future capacity to behave socially. (Gerhardt 2004: 210)

She does point out that this can all sound quite 'daunting' and that in fact, most parents 'do this anyway'. Yet the implications, according to the *Mothering Magazine* article, are profound:

What this means for parents raising children in today's world is sweeping. We need cultural changes – changes in expectation, in our view of parents, in our definitions of feminism and masculinity, in our economic systems and medical understandings. In its broader applications, attachment theory requires us to rethink most of what our society has taught us. We must let go of old learning and erroneous information in order to re-attune to our own connective instincts. (Porter 2003)

Advocates of scheduled feeding and sleeping routines can thus be 'shunned', according to the article, because their methods have been 'proven' to be detrimental to infant development.

'The Science'

The intention here is not to question the validity of this scientific research as such. Rather, it is to think about the social life of science – not so much practices of fact-making (Latour and Woolgar 1986), but rather scientific authority within contemporary parenting debates. When 'science' says something is healthiest for infants, it has the effect of shutting down debate; that is, it dictates what parents should do. Yet whilst science tells us much about the world, the meaning we ascribe to these 'facts' (i.e., how we should act on them) is hardly straightforward.

Furedi (2008) has remarked that the replacement of scientific evidence with a more generic 'Science' is a trend on the increase. Certainly, infant feeding and parenting policy is increasingly 'evidence-based':

[T]oday, it frequently seems as if scientific authority is replacing religious and moral authority, and in the process being transformed into a dogma.... Parents are advised to adopt this or that child-rearing technique on the grounds that 'the research' has shown what is best for kids. Scientific studies are frequently used to instruct people on how to conduct their relationships and family life, and on what food they should eat, how much alcohol they should drink, how frequently they can expose their skin to the sun, and even how they should have sex. Virtually every aspect of human life is discussed in scientific terms, and justified with reference to a piece of research or by appealing to the judgment of experts. (Furedi 2008)

Furedi's argument echoes long-standing concerns about the dangers of blurring the line between description and prescription. In the eighteenth century David Hume counselled, in his *Treatise Concerning Human Nature*:

> In every system of morality, which I have hitherto met with, I have always remark'd, that the author proceeds for some time in the ordinary ways of reasoning, and establishes the being of a God, or makes observations concerning human affairs; when all of a sudden I am surpriz'd to find, that instead of the usual copulations of propositions, *is*, and *is not*, I meet with no proposition that is not connected with an *ought*, or an *ought not*. This change is imperceptible; but is however, of the last consequence. For as this *ought*, or *ought not*, expresses some new relation or affirmation, 'tis necessary that it shou'd be observ'd and explain'd; and at the same time that a reason should be given; for what seems altogether inconceivable, how this new relation can be a deduction from others, which are entirely different from it. (Hume 2000, Section 1, Book 3)

Hume's is-ought distinction remains pertinent today because parenting is not only an exercise in creating scientifically optimal children: '[T]urning science into an arbiter of policy and behaviour only serves to confuse matters. ... Yes, the search for truth requires scientific experimentation and the discovery of new facts; but it also demands answers about the *meaning* of those facts, and those answers can only be clarified through moral, philosophical investigation and debate' (Furedi 2008). The gap between description (what is healthiest, however defined) and prescription (what should be done) is particularly relevant for parenting practices that stretch over a period of years: one accountability strategy mothers provided as to why they had planned to, and continued to, breastfeed their children was that long-term breastfeeding was what 'science says is best'.

Apple (1995) has described the ideology of scientific motherhood as one that designates good mothers as those who are guided by scientific information, subjugating their own perspectives to authoritative experts (Hausman 2003: 3). Similarly, the ideology of intensive motherhood celebrates scientifically informed care (Hays 1996). Although Apple talks specifically about the almost wholesale shift from breastfeeding to bottle-feeding in the twentieth-century United States, based on offering a 'scientific, modern' form of feeding, her insights might just as well be applied to this new generation of 'neuroscientific motherhood'. Today, this kind of science – seen as a battle against the 'scientisation' of the formula manufacturers Apple describes – has been given the extra twist of 'returning to nature' rather than moving away from it.

This reliance on science is problematic when 'science' becomes a yardstick by which we outline appropriate human interactions. 'Science' has the capacity to flatten out the affective, joyous qualities of the parenting relationship. Maternal love, according to the title of Gerhardt's book, is no longer simply an enjoyable part of the parenting experience, but also a tool for optimising brain development. As Hausman (2003) comments about the use of science in breastfeeding advocacy more widely:

> Breastfeeding advocacy, while resting partially on the idea of maternal nursing as natural mothering, most often looks to science to verify its value and promote its interests. Such advocacy is problematic, I think, when it relies increasingly on the scientific case in its favour because that reliance simply knits a complex biosocial practice ever more firmly into science as the final arbiter of what we, as humans, should eat, how we should sleep, what kind of relationship we should develop with our children, and so on. (Hausman 2003: 152)

This is particularly problematic where doing what is 'best' requires considerable work (and/or socio-economic ability) on the part of the mother: such flattening can eclipse areas of the infant feeding and parenting relationship, to the extent that other demands on a mother's time are left in the shade. This is perhaps particularly pertinent where 'science says' that intensive, embodied nurture carried out by the mother is the optimal form of care.

'The Science' and 'Informed Choice'

The use of scientific evidence about infant feeding is typical in LLL texts and in meeting presentations, where the *Womanly Art of Breastfeeding* or *The Breastfeeding Answer Book* were often consulted. Information derived from research is the basis on which parents are expected to make an 'informed choice' about how they raise their children. On the whole, my respondents tended to see women who do not breastfeed for long periods of time as victims: subject to marketing by rapacious formula manufacturers; 'let down' by a health service that does not provide them accurate information about, and support for, breastfeeding; and bound into inflexible working contracts.

Certainly, women lamented that health professionals, who were supposed to educate mothers, were 'totally ignorant' (Virginia), and remarkably often I heard tales of health professionals who appeared to have little or no knowledge of the basic lactation process:

Lauren [*42, breastfeeding her 2½-year-old daughter*]: Once, I had this young [doctor] who said 'Oh my god! You are still breastfeeding! That is fantastic … but do you still have milk?!' And I said, no, I have coca-cola! … I mean! It makes you wonder. And I said to him, you know, it is your job to be telling women they should breastfeed, as a doctor, as a paediatrician! And I don't know, I have just been shocked by how little doctors and paediatricians know about breastfeeding.

These comments echo the work of Rose and Novas (2004) on 'expert patients', who appropriate (scientific) knowledge as a means of self-realisation. Indeed, many of the women interviewed had encyclopaedic knowledge about breastfeeding and felt that health professionals were severely lacking in this area:

Sandra [*Leader, 35, breastfeeding her 4-year-old daughter*]: We are often told that breast milk has no nutritional value after a year old, which is rubbish … I work a lot with health professionals, and I know that they only have one day [of] training on this, sometimes taught by a rep from a formula company. *One day*! You are lucky if you find a GP or a health visitor who has any extra info on it at all. I have done about three and a half years of reading, I have had fifteen months of training, I am always reading up on it … to be accredited as a leader. It is one of our responsibilities. So, I know more than most breastfeeding professionals, but they have the status – they get paid.

LLL exists in part to fill this gap, and league leaders were very clear that the purpose of the group is to provide people with 'information, not advice', with the implication that information has 'no emotional content':

Jemima [*Chair of Council*]: One of the things you will find between LLL and the other organizations is that we do not give advice, we give information and support. We [says forcefully] *do not give* advice – that is hammered home in our training; we give information and support. We meet people wherever they are in their breastfeeding relationship and experience. That is where we will meet them and offer them the support that they need to deal with where they are at the time … we are not a proselytising or evangelising organisation.

LLL leaders passionately disagree with any notion that they 'force' their ideas upon mothers, making them feel guilty if they do not choose to breastfeed and continue breastfeeding until the child outgrows the need. Giving women 'real' information – such as that derived from scientific studies[6] – is seen to be a means of empowering them by offering an informed choice. Should mothers feel guilty about not having breastfed to full term, either now or in the past, this information offers them the chance to change their choices in the future:

> *Jemima [Chair of Council]*: I think that people that feel guilty need to reassure themselves that they never wanted to do the worst for their baby, they wanted the best for their baby, and they must have made choices ... based on the information they had at the time, and what was right for them and their family. If they have subsequently found other ways of doing things, then again they are free to make changes.... And that does not need to be with any recriminations. Because we are a learning mammal, and are able to look at a situation with different things; we learn things ... and so 'with this information I can react in this way.'

Thus some LLL leaders understand guilt as a positively useful emotion for women to feel – if it spurs them to act in a different way.[7] One anglophone leader in France compared giving women information about the benefits of breastfeeding to the campaign against tobacco and alcohol use:

> *Chloe [Long-serving anglophone leader, emphasis added]*: Does it make people feel guilty? This is very important in France. People will feel guilty, if they have something to feel guilty about. Doctors will tell women not to drink, and not to smoke, as it is very dangerous for the baby, if it is a smoker or someone who drinks, are they not going to not tell them?! They'll tell them. They can't control what she does outside. She may continue to smoke, and drink, and she may feel guilty. That's her choice. To feel guilty.
>
> And breastfeeding is in a way the same thing. It is not an instance where you cannot give real information. Is it to make them feel guilty? No. Is it to make them feel bad? No. *If they do feel bad about it, that's their choice, what they do with it. It is to give information, and to give them a choice* ... and in the teaching department we have a very *clear* approach in how you give information. *Information has no emotional content to it.* 'The studies show that there is less hospitalisation amongst breastfed babies,' you can agree or disagree and feel guilty or not, but these are the facts. What we find is that people who did not breastfeed are very angry that they were not told. They are furious. And it doesn't matter if it's at age 60. They are furious at finding out they were not helped. *If a woman goes away feeling guilty, that's her problem. She has the option to change her behaviour.*

In this case, Chloe is talking about breastfeeding in general, rather than full-term feeding, yet the point is well made: for her, guilt is something a mother can 'choose'. LLL recognises that some breast-feeding counsellors 'can find it difficult to remain objective'. The *Leader's Handbook* states:

> Some breastfeeding counsellors find it difficult to remain objective when they strongly disagree with a mother's choices [for example, to mix-feed their children]. When feelings run high, it can be helpful to remember that your primary purpose is to act as a sounding board for the mother. To effectively fulfil this purpose, personal opinions, feelings, and experiences need to be kept in the background, keeping the mother as the main focus. The counsellor's job is to help the mother clarify her own feelings and offer information and options that will help her make an informed choice. (LLLI 2003: 10)

Despite the discourse of choice then, wherever long-term breast-feeding and attachment parenting are deemed scientifically best for children, an intensive motherhood framework dictates that 'good mothers' will be attachment mothers. There is clearly a 'right' and a 'wrong' choice here. For those who do not (or cannot) make the 'right' choice, there is potential for guilt and judgement, by oneself or others, for failing at the tasks of 'good' mothering (Knaak 2006).

This is evident in the way Amelia talks about people who *have* been 'educated' about the benefits of breastfeeding and still do not breastfeed, whom she terms 'wilfully ignorant':

> *Amelia [33, breastfeeding her almost-3-year-old son, emphasis added]*: [T]here are a lot of stay at home mums, for example, in [my area], but who don't see the value in breastfeeding for any length of time … and I think, *that reaches the level of a wilful ignorance at some point.* You are better focusing your efforts on *people who haven't made an informed choice to be ignorant.*

As a full-term breastfeeder talking about why other mothers did not breastfeed, Amelia said that she felt 'like a genius on a planet of idiots'. Felicity, writing about her 'extended' feeding, said in the questionnaire:

> *Questionnaire*: Do you feel that you have to explain your decisions about how you feed your infant(s) to other people?
>
> *Felicity [33, 12-year-old daughter, just-weaned 2-year-old son]*: Yes
>
> *Questionnaire*: Please say a little more, and how this makes you feel, as a mother:
>
> *Felicity*: I'm educated enough now about the issues not to give a damn what others think … ignorant, status quo following puppets … plus

I'm not English so I'm used to people judging me for my 'different' ways of doing things.

Questionnaire: What is your most common reaction to being judged over your decisions [to continue breastfeeding]?

Felicity: Fight back with 'did you know...' interesting research, facts, stories ... my decision is evidence based and theirs [those who do not breastfeed into toddlerhood] is not. Then again, I'm really well read on this stuff now. I'm super empowered with the knowledge I have.

The benefits of breastfeeding and attachment parenting serve as a (seemingly) morally neutral canon that mothers can apply to defend their mothering choices and 'spread the word' about appropriate parenting to both new mothers attending the group and members of wider society. For certain women, sharing 'information' with other mothers, either on a one-to-one basis or through the more formalised activism described earlier, was a source of great enjoyment – as the woman in the quote above puts it, she is 'super empowered' by the knowledge that she has gleaned at LLL and through her own reading. Any criticisms she has of other women are depersonalised, because science 'has no emotional content'. In this case, science appears to be less about understanding than about belief, as this meeting observation indicates:

A mother describes how she responds to those who criticise her decision to breastfeed her son until his seventh birthday, by saying: 'I mean, do you want to see studies? Because I can show you studies!' There are laughs and cheers from the rest of the group.

At meetings, it was not unusual to hear mothers – generally the 'core of the core' – speak quite vocally and critically about mothers who do not parent their children in ways akin to attachment parenting. Often, this was done very forcefully, though LLL leaders were keen to temper any 'over-zealous converts' (whom the leader Janet described as 'more LLL than LLL').

Conclusion

As the cow goddess cartoon and comments in the introduction highlight, some contradictions inhere in the use of 'science' to bolster arguments around attachment parenting. On the one hand, 'a reasoned and measured response is not what the situation calls for', and mothers do 'what feels right in their hearts'. On the other, there is a notion that science should be the ultimate arbiter in decision-making around infant feeding. Calling for 'more research', one mother, writing in the comments, says:

> **Laura** said, February 3, 2008 @ 7:56 am Some of what Charlotte wrote is true. There is little support (e.g., alloparents) for nurturing children the AP way in modern industrialized countries.... [But] just because humans invented something doesn't mean it's a good solution. Maybe Charlotte should entertain the notion that women involved in breastfeeding are actually adapting to *something,* and then she should figure out what that is. Are extreme breastfeeders in fact early adapters? Or are [we] just fringe radicals struggling with outcast-identity issues?... Her observations are constrained by what she knows, and she's probably some smart young 20-something getting her doctorate at Cambridge who can only rely on what science tells her (until she experiences childrearing firsthand). There is no evidence that children in the industrialized world who are raised AP-style are better off than peers who were breastfed for one year but otherwise were birthed by c-section, transported in strollers, and placed in cribs. Indeed, I know plenty of perfectly wonderful mothers with great kids who did the latter. We need more research.

It would be wrong to imply that the attachment mothers I worked with saw science in isolation from 'evolution' or 'affect' – certainly, 'science' appeared as the earliest accountability strategy, being understood as the most robust. Yet the next chapter, which explores the affective dimension of women's accountability strategies, argues that this aspect is, in fact, intimately tied up with their decision-making.

Notes

1. For an interesting discussion on this topic see 'When proof is not proof,' retrieved 27 April 2009 from http://mainstreamparenting.wordpress.com/2008/01/23/when-proof-is-not-proof-apnp-research/ See also Eyer (1992).
2. The link to Prescott's work, retrieved 5 June 2008, should actually read http://www.violence.de/prescott/ttf/article.html
3. The reference here is to Schore (2001).
4. References in this paragraph are to Schore (2001), Bowlby (1969) and Spangler et al. (1994).
5. References in this paragraph are to Tronick and Weinberg (1997), Perry et al. (1995), Schore (2001) and McEwen (2000).
6. As opposed to information with a profit agenda, from formula milk manufacturers.

7. Conversely, one leader noted that helping women to wean was one way LLL helps mothers deal with 'guilt':

> *Sandra [Leader, 35, breastfeeding her 4-year-old daughter]*: I really resent that idea that LLL puts pressure on women to breastfeed, or forces women to breastfeed. A lot of what we do is about telling women 'how to stop' without causing them or their baby damage or too much pain. For example, one woman I talked to about stopping felt a lot better having discussed all the options, not guilty about not 'giving the best shot', and that is a big part of it. If they stop it is because they really want to.

Chapter 8

'WHAT FEELS RIGHT IN MY HEART'

HORMONES, MORALITY AND AFFECTIVE BREASTFEEDING

Throughout this research, it has been a struggle to write about what, for many women, is the most important accountability strategy in their narratives of full-term breastfeeding: say what you like about nature and science, this simply 'feels right'. Writing about the intimate, affective dimension of breastfeeding has been particularly difficult because many women found their feelings, especially about breastfeeding their older children, hard to verbalise – as something almost *beyond* expression. Many said simply, 'You just know it's the right thing to do. You'll know too when you have children of your own' (Virginia).

This, of course, poses problems for the researcher. Arguably, everything in parenting is affect-based, which makes 'choices' both passionate and personal. For other authors, putting personal experience into academic framework is the typical remedy: 'I am an academic by trade and a mother by vocation. ... I have known for a long time that bodies are representations, performing elaborate rituals of signification even in the their most intimate moments; what I came to know from breastfeeding my daughter is that these ritual performances originate in flesh that is overdetermined but still miraculous' (Sutherland 1999: 1).

Yet as a woman without children, I have no experiential anecdotes to draw on in my understandings or descriptions of breastfeeding. Earlier, I argued that my lack of experience was useful, as it allowed me to step, to some extent, outside the otherwise fraught arena of intensive motherhood and infant feeding, affording a useful research space. But it obviously has its shortcomings: as an anthropologist, how can one write on the basis of only observation, not 'participation' – particularly in a practice so central to this text?

Women would talk about 'doing what feels right in my heart'; a phrase that resists collapsing into either the bodily or the moral domain (on this, see also Tomori 2010). In this chapter I attempt to pay due respect to the intensity of feeling that breastfeeding generates (whilst also appreciating that these feelings may not be confined to breastfeeding, as many mothers who formula feed will attest). I do this through a theoretical framework of 'affect' (Clough and Halley 2007; Connolly 1999) that enables consideration of both of bodies (nipples and mouths) and morals (what women believe to be the right thing to do).

Because of the Hormones: 'It Feels Right'

It was typical to hear women describe their experiences of breastfeeding with reference to the hormones involved in the process, and in turn, the feelings that these were understood to generate. Generally, they echoed the language used by La Leche League and the attachment parenting community more broadly. In *The Womanly Art of Breastfeeding*, LLL states:

Breastfeeding hormones
Niles Newton, a psychologist who was a long-time friend and advisor to La Leche League, described oxytocin, the hormone that triggers the let-down reflex, as 'the hormone of love'. Oxytocin triggers nurturing behaviour, which in Dr Newton's words, is 'an essential ingredient in the success of reproduction'. Both prolactin and oxytocin may help to produce the feelings of relaxation that mothers come to associate with nursing sessions. Many women recognise that they feel calmer during the months they are nursing their babies and better able to cope with whatever comes along. A recent study showed that lactation suppresses the nervous system's hormonal response to stress. Nature intends for mothers to enjoy breastfeeding their babies, and the good feelings that come with breastfeeding help mothers become more attached to their babies. (LLLI 2004 375–376)

The term hormone was first introduced by Starling in 1905 to refer to chemical messengers in the bloodstream. The account by LLL uses it in an evolutionary paradigm: tuning in to the chemical messengers enables women to enjoy motherhood because of the feelings they induce (relaxation, love), which in turn makes for more attached, better mothers.

In previous chapters, I noted the tendency to link our understandings of appropriate maternal behaviour too closely to 'what science says is best', or indeed, to 'what nature intended'; similarly, it should not be simply assumed that if one has high levels of oxytocin in the body one does/should feel motherly and nurturing. This is not to ignore the feelings of a breastfeeding woman, or her child. Quite the opposite: it is to suggest that the feelings of 'love' a mother feels during breastfeeding are not simply the effects of oxytocin. Paying attention only to the material basis of feelings, expressed in the language of hormones, risks belittling them, much as saying feelings of irritability, sadness or frustration in the premenstrual period are 'hormonal' can seem to dismiss them. Feelings might well be influenced by fluctuating levels of progestin and oestrogen, but this makes little difference in how one actually *feels* – one is still happy, or sad. In this regard, explaining the 'is' has little instrumental effect – save to bracket these feelings into the 'normal' range of a female physiology, which is in itself a political statement.

This chapter therefore looks more closely at how attachment mothers spoke about breastfeeding 'feeling' right – as an accountability strategy to justify their non-normative parenting practices – not only through idioms of bodily materiality but more broadly in terms of affectivity and morality.

Affective Breastfeeding

A recent wave of scholarship has urged greater attention to the 'affective' lives of our informants (Clough and Halley 2007; Connolly 1999; Massumi 2002b). This favours the more traditional attention to 'emotions' that, these scholars argue, has become too loaded a term – not least because it replicates long-held distinctions of mind/body, head/heart and so forth. Furthermore, whilst I have found much of this work useful, I am not preoccupied with one of its central questions, concerning the rationality (or otherwise) of emotions. To cite Ducey (2007):

> The concept of affect as I use it refers to a different register of phenomena than the concept of emotions, at least as the latter term is

usually used in sociology. The necessity of holding a distinction between emotions and affect is supported by research and thought in a number of fields such as philosophy, neuroscience, and communication studies. The neuroscientist Antonio Damasio recently proposed a distinction between emotions and feelings, though I propose to call the same distinction that between affect and emotions. (Ducey 2007: 190)

Ducey's argument, drawing heavily on Damasio, is that 'emotion' in the social sciences has taken for granted the relationship between stimulus and response (see also Jenkins and Valiente 1994). He prefers to separate out the process, which I have found useful when dealing with accounts of breastfeeding being 'inexpressible'. Damasio (2006 shows that when an organism encounters a stimulus able to trigger an emotional response, 'emotion' consists in the first part of an organism's physical response ('affect'), mapped and modified by the brain. This is not necessarily a conscious process, since affects 'are modifications of the body that are autonomous from conscious thought and attention' (Ducey 2007: 190). Emotions are 'largely constituted by the perception of a bodily state', or the 'perception of the body state forms the essence of a feeling' (Damasio 2006: 55 and 89, in Ducey 2007: 190). Thus emotions require a level of awareness, based on mental maps of the body's physical state (affect). This need not be a linear progression from one to the other, the emotions we feel being equally influenced by experience and memory. Indeed, how affect becomes emotion is the gap of interest to the researcher. And because affect may be expressed as emotion in variable, culturally patterned ways, anthropological engagement is particularly warranted here.

Simply put, then, 'affect' is the preconscious response to a stimulus (e.g., mouth on nipple, or a let-down reflex), not necessarily expressed or verbalised in the language of 'emotion'. There is therefore a trap here, in trying to describe the affective element of breastfeeding through the narrations of my informants:

> ... language only captures what has emerged from the level of intensity, that affect cannot be exposed through language. The conscious statements by people interviewed in ... research are not representations of what has happened in affect, but rather, indications of the significance for the organism or system of what has happened in affect. The discourse that emerged in these interviews as a particularly charged indication of changes in affect is that of 'meaning'. (Ducey 2007: 192–193)

Yet this framework is useful here *because* of the accounts women give about breastfeeding as indescribable yet significant:[1]

Questionnaire: How would you describe breastfeeding your child?

Amelia [*33, breastfeeding her almost-3-year-old son*]: Indescribable to me, but an oasis of calm.

Jane [*Leader applicant, 25, breastfeeding her 16-month-old son*]: Too amazing to begin to even describe.

It seems that for many women the sensations breastfeeding generates both remain at a physical, pre-verbalised level ('indescribable') and later go on to form the basis of love (a reflexive emotion). Separating emotion from affect here is therefore a useful device, even if only heuristically:

Charlotte: So what does it feel like? Is it nice?

Lauren [*42, breastfeeding her 2½-year-old daughter*]: Well at the beginning, it really helps your uterus get back into shape, so you can really feel the contractions, you know. [*Aside, to her child*: Booby? What's that (child's nickname)? You want booby? Ok, come here. Booby yes, booby booby booby!] So yes, at the beginning you feel these contractions.... And erm, I think it is more psychological now, it's that I can feed and nurture my baby with what my body is producing. And actually, I read an article about mothers' milk the other day [in *The Ecologist*], and they still don't know what it contains.

Charlotte: Yeah.

Lauren: It's amazing. And I am sure there are some things on the subtle level you can't prove scientifically ... maybe love, who knows?

'Affect' is necessarily relational, which makes it a particularly appropriate framework for discussing breastfeeding – a symbiotic process, involving an emergent double subjectivity (of the mother and the child):

By 'affect' I don't mean 'emotion' in the everyday sense. The way I use it comes primarily from Spinoza. He talks of the body in terms of its capacity for *affecting* or being *affected*. These two are not different capacities – they always go together. When you affect something, you are at the same time opening yourself up to being affected in turn, and in a slightly different way than you might have been the moment before. You have made a transition, however slight.... A body is defined by what capacities it carries from step to step. What these are exactly is changing constantly. A body's ability to affect or be affected – its charge of affect – isn't something fixed. (Massumi 2002b: 212–213)

The comfort that *both* mother and child receive in the process of breastfeeding was certainly something my informants talked of as a mutual endeavour, one that was particularly poignant in the pre-verbal stage. Many mothers are comforted by being able to comfort their children, despite not knowing exactly what it is they want.[2] Valerie echoes this reciprocal benefit when she writes of breastfeeding as being 'embraced in love':

> *Questionnaire*: Was it important for you to feed your child at the breast?
>
> *Valerie [33, breastfeeding her 11-month-old son]*: Yes.
>
> *Questionnaire*: Please say why:
>
> *Valerie*: Important for us to bond. A natural feeling and emotion to be close and embraced in love while nursing. So I could just sit and watch the baby and fall in love with him. Base human emotion of protecting and doing the best for him.

Instinct and Intuition: Some Contradictions

For many women, breastfeeding was the 'obvious' thing to do, in that it was spurred by intense 'gut feelings' (e.g., the 'base human emotion of protecting' in Valerie's quote):

> *Questionnaire*: Why was it important to feed your child with breast milk?
>
> *Signe [Leader applicant, 30, breastfeeding her 3-year-old son]*: Felt like the natural and obvious thing to do, I didn't even really consider an alternative.

Many attachment mothers spoke about this importance as 'instinctual' (and it is typical to read in attachment parenting books that this form of parenting is simply a matter of 'following one's instincts'). The implication here is that women have universal and in-built mothering urges with which they simply need to get in touch. Those who lack these instincts (arguably those who use bottles, instead of feeding at the breast) are regarded as having been failed by the necessary support mechanisms, or as not yet 'in tune' with their own bodies. Claudine, a young French woman living in London with her boyfriend, expressed such considerations:

> *Questionnaire*: Do you think that women are under pressure to feed their infants in a certain way at certain times?

Claudine [*24, breastfeeding her 17-month-old daughter, emphasis added*]:
Not me personally but I can understand how other women might
feel pressured to bottle-feed (for a 'relief' night out, or if the baby's
weight isn't following the chart ...) Also I understand some women
feel under pressure to start solids whether their baby is ready or not,
or to stop breastfeeding their older babies/toddlers because it is not
'normal'. And also I have recently heard that some women feel 'pressured into breastfeeding' because of all the 'hype'. It is my own very
personal opinion that a woman who really doesn't want to breastfeed
either doesn't truly appreciate the risks of formula-feeding, or if she
does then must have some serious unresolved issues about her body.
*Sorrrrryy but I still cannot really understand how a mother could not want
to feed her own baby.* Surely, only a pretty f***ed up society can create
such problems ...

The implication is that breastfeeding is natural for women, and
that women, as a universal category, have an inherent capacity to
breastfeed and to enjoy breastfeeding. The discourse reflects an understanding of maternal love and natural motherhood as expressed
through breastfeeding: it is said to continue the special relationship
women had with their infants in the womb as an extension of the
natural, embodied and intimate connection begun in pregnancy –
indeed, many mothers referred to it as 'the fourth trimester'.

The rosy picture of breastfeeding as something enjoyable and
easy, at which mothers should be able to succeed, is not reflected
in the actual experience of many women who have major problems
in the postpartum period. This was certainly the case during fieldwork I conducted in a central London hospital, where breastfeeding
seemed far from natural for many of the mothers I met. As Wall puts
it, 'Having encountered unexpected difficulties, and eventually giving up on breastfeeding, women report feeling isolated and unique
and feeling as though their bodies have failed and as though they
have failed as mothers in a fundamental way' (Wall 2001: 598).
On this front, much breastfeeding literature acknowledges that it
is 'perfectly normal' to have some difficulties with breastfeeding,
though these are generally characterised as small concerns, reme-
diable by seeking the advice of a health professional – or by being
motivated and keeping a sense of humour.

Talking about instinct is highly problematic when it comes to
human beings, as it implies some sort of involuntary response,
or mindless activity, sometimes witnessed amongst other animals
(Mainstream Parenting Resources 2008).[3] It would be unwise, then,
to use affect as simply a label for something automatic, instinctive or

hard-wired and therefore 'natural'. Human parenting is a far more complex endeavour. Massumi (2002a), in conversation with Zournazi, counsels against this too:

> *Zournazi*: Is affect primal?
>
> *Massumi*: I wouldn't say it's primal, if that means more 'natural'. I don't think affective intensity is any more natural than the ability to stand back and reflect on something, or the ability to pin something down in language. But I guess it might be considered primal in the sense that it is direct. (Massumi 2002a: 215)

And it would be unfair to suggest that the informants here have so simplistic a view of instinct – that is, of mother love as something automatic or unthinking. Indeed, these women are highly reflexive about it. Women more typically talked about 'doing what feels right in my heart'. In this case *intuition*, not instinct, might be a more appropriate way of talking about these sensations. Thus Pippa, a long-serving LLL leader, says that the LLL philosophy was like finding 'something I felt in my heart all along, but couldn't actually articulate'.

Ways of Knowing

Robbie Davis-Floyd and Elizabeth Davis (1997) write in defence of intuition as a way of knowing in their article 'Intuition as Authoritative Knowledge in Midwifery and Home Birth'. They stress certain characteristics of intuition: confidence in the process, a sense of certainty or truth, the suddenness and immediacy of the knowledge, the association of intuition with insight, and the 'preverbal' nature of the knowledge. They argue that intuition as a knowledge practice has been devalued in contemporary American society, which is dominated by a technocratic model. Drawing on Martin (1987), they point out that mechanistic metaphors for the universe and body have gained importance since the time of Descartes: 'Conscious deductive reasoning, which can be logically explained and replicated, is the most machine like form of thought' (Davis-Floyd and Davis 1997: 318). Intuition, by contrast, is a deep cognitive process *without* conscious awareness.

As human beings, argue Davis-Floyd and Davis, we use both forms of reasoning, so to ignore intuition (or, affect) is to see only half of the picture. In the context of reproductive health, and specifically birth, they argue that machines are more commonly understood as the source of 'authoritative knowledge' (a concept originally developed by Bridgette Jordan in 1978[4]). Although relying on a rather problematic nature/culture : good/bad split – as in the case of 'some women in the United States who supervalue nature and their natural bodies over science and technology' (Davis-Floyd and Davis 1997: 316) – the point is well made that intuitive knowledge is not valued in contemporary debates about birth and parenting. Indeed, as argued in Chapter 1, parents are increasingly told not to trust their own instincts but rather to follow the advice of a parenting expert, who then advises on which instinct to tune in to. Davis-Floyd and Davis quote one midwife who says:

> I think, because we are in a culture that doesn't respect intuition, and has a very narrow definition of knowledge, we can get caught into the trap of that narrowness. Intuition is another kind of knowledge – deeply embodied. It's not up there in the stars. It *is* knowing, just as much as intellectual knowing. It's not fluff, which is what the culture tries to do with it. *Judy Luce, Homebirth midwife.* (Davis-Floyd and Davis 1997: 317)[5]

Whilst intuition might be a midwife's guide, for the first-time mother it can be problematic as a 'way of knowing' because intuition is actually the result of past experiences. Klein, a cognitive psychologist who studies intuition, shows that it manifests itself through subconscious thought processes, and that the more experience one has with the topic, the likelier one is to be able to intuit appropriate behaviour (Klein 1998). He cites the example of nurses in a neonatal ward working with babies who sometimes develop a septic condition that can rapidly kill them unless action is taken. Researchers heard many stories of nurses who would glance at an infant and instantly recognise their need for treatment. When asked how they knew, nurses would respond by saying 'you just know'. They understand this 'knowing' as intuition, yet the more accurate answer would be recognition: in interviews, the nurses narrated subtle yet important clues to an infant's septic infection (greying colour, frequent crying followed by listlessness, etc.).

If intuition is (at least in part) the result of past experience, this obviously has profound implications for how we understand it in descriptions of parenting, and particularly mothering. Given that people have different experiences (or no experience) of parenting, as well as a wide range of intimate relationships, it stands to reason that they will have different 'intuitive messages' about the appropriate way to parent – which makes 'tuning into your instincts' or 'following your intuition' a problematic accountability strategy for attachment parents.

Agency When You 'Just Know'

During research it seemed that many attachment mothers 'just knew' that what they were doing was right – in many senses it was a decision seemingly based not on thought, but on instinct or intuition, reifying the body consciousness that is so central to the philosophy (Bobel 2002: 91). For all their reflexivity about their parenting choices, we might more accurately say that it was a process of reflection on a (selected) predetermination – the predetermination that nature, confirmed by science, knows best.

A typical trope in women's accounts was that of having made a mothering 'journey', whereby truths about mothering, which are always known, deep inside mothers, are 'revealed' to women – often through contact with LLL members, and through information that helped them 'tune in' to their inner natures. Attachment mothers would talk about coming to their current positions through a series of 'epiphanies' (Bobel [2002] also recognised this). 'Before' they were more mainstream; now, having become informed, they have 'realised' the path they wanted to take. There was therefore a separation from mothers who 'hadn't yet made this journey'. One leader said, talking about her work:

> Annette [Leader, breastfeeding her 7-year-old son]: I have gone down a particular path, because I have realised certain things about motherhood. I've helped mothers who are on a similar path to me, but I can't necessarily help those mothers who are on a different path to me, or don't think the same way as me. They don't necessarily want, or are able, to hear what I have to say.

But this is not to say that it was something felt statically and uniformly by all women. Many of the women had planned on going back to work soon after their baby's birth but were shocked to find they did not want to. Some were surprised at how their consciousness changed as they became mothers. One woman talked about how shocked she was that she would 'fall in love' with her baby:

> Chloe [Long-standing anglophone Leader]: Yeah. I mean I had never planned on staying at home with my child. I had a full-time job, I

was going to go back, and I did. And I quit two weeks later. It wasn't
easy to make that decision. It never occurred to me that I would quit.
You know, that I would fall in love with this baby, that just wasn't
part of the plan. You know, I was going to pump my milk – by hand,
as there were no pumps yet. ... But I just couldn't bear it. I couldn't
bear leaving him.

Bobel terms these narratives 'shock-shift' stories, since the shock
of this feeling usually engenders changed behaviour. Interestingly,
the choice between career and family comes down to being 'no
choice', when rationalised and accounted for in terms of doing what
'feels right'. Any intellectual sense of what things should be like is
overridden by how things 'really' are. The body determines social
practice and sends messages in the forms of 'gut feelings' (Bobel
2002: 95). Once one makes this discovery, there is no going back. To
take Bobel's argument:

> If we listen to their narratives of self-motivated decisions to quit jobs
> and careers and stay at home full-time with babies, we see strong,
> self-determined women who actively choose a particular lifestyle,
> even if that lifestyle denies the individual mother's self-actualisation.
> But if we listen a bit more closely, tuning into their motivations to
> mother in this particular way, a different picture comes into focus. ...
> Natural mothers ... may actively embrace the 'nature is best' ideology,
> but once they become attached to this ideology – buying into it com-
> pletely without regret – they surrender their capacity to make choices
> and in some ways become passive objects. (Bobel 2002: 97–98)

For Bobel, the 'nature is best' ideology is taken on to such an
extent that it reaches hegemonic proportions, transforming women
into individuals who surrender their own agency for the sake of
their family. If, she argues, an agent is a 'conscious, rational subject. ... acting in their own interest', the accounts of 'natural' mothers (with whom she worked in the US) are troubling: 'Rather than
thinking through their options as parents, they draw their insight
from feelings that cannot be explained or reasoned' (Bobel 2002:
98). Theoretically, these women could choose to parent 'like everyone else' – but even as they speak of choice, they speak of being guided by a feeling that cannot be disputed: nature knows best.
Natural mothering is the only 'real' choice. All other choices flow
from this most fundamental one. The rhetoric of science, used to
describe these decisions, appears to validate this choice as one that
is informed. For Bobel, however, it is an acceptance of an ideology of
biology-as-destiny; 'choice' is undermined by 'just knowing'.

I take a slightly more sympathetic view. In the light of the highly accountable arena of contemporary parenting, discussed in previous chapters, handing over responsibility for one's child-rearing to some grander narrative (of the natural, the scientific, or even instinct) can provide women with a sort of relief from the constant requirement of accountability. Each of these strategies, albeit in different ways, forecloses further probing.

I also wonder whether Bobel's critique might have the effect of invalidating the maternal experience – once again, pointing to tensions within feminist discourses. If one cannot argue for something simply on the basis that it 'feels right,' does that not leave us in something of a sad state when it comes to other issues such as what sorts of things we like to eat, our sleeping habits or even our sexual preferences? Bobel's problem, presumably, concerns the point at which description becomes prescription, where women who do not 'tune in' to their 'instincts' are cast as somehow substandard mothers. Here, I experiment by arguing for a defence of affective knowledge – things that we 'know in our heart' – as a valid accountability strategy in parenting, as much as in other areas of personal life.

A Moral Good?

I want to consider this as a question of morality. When women talk about breastfeeding 'feeling right,' they do not mean it in a physical sense alone. Breastfeeding is certainly an affective and emotional commitment to their child, but at the same time, it is something they believe to be *right*:

> *Questionnaire*: Do you think that women are under pressure to feed their infants in a certain way at certain times?
>
> *Claire* [*38, mother of a 7-year-old son, breastfeeding her 11-month-old son*]: Yes
>
> *Questionnaire*: If yes; please say how so, and how this has influenced your own experiences:
>
> *Claire*: It felt right to breastfeed, but there are so many pressures to conform to the FF [formula feeding] brigade, which I was not willing to do.... [I] felt very strongly [that I ought] to breastfeed, and give babies the best start.

In response to the second question, Virginia wrote:

Virginia [24, breastfeeding her 17-month-old daughter]: I can't explain it,
but you just know that it's the right thing to do. I don't know how I
know, but I do. It's just something I feel so strongly. You'll know too
when you have your own children.

Bobel would dismiss these accounts as something beyond intel-
lectualisation, and therefore invalid as an accountability strategy. In
this, I suggest she has made what Damasio (2006) would refer to as
'Descartes' Error': that is, she has separated reason (which she validates) from feeling (which, being based on un-verbalisable bodily
messages, she does not; although it's worth noting here that Descartes himself was not necessarily giving a description of how human beings are, but a reflection of society's values and modes of
operation). Here, women are validating a moral choice on the basis
of feeling: I want to see how far we can take this as an accountability
strategy. My argument mirrors that of Davis-Floyd and Davis, to the
extent that I validate 'ways of knowing' other than the 'rational',
albeit with a different intention.

Damasio (2006) argues that throughout Western philosophical
thought since the time of Descartes, there has been a separation
within the subject of the mind from the body, and therefore of reason from emotion (which, following Ducey, have been separated
into the different elements of affect and emotion here). For Descartes, control of our 'passions' through reason was what made us
human, distinct from the rest of the animal kingdom. Damasio's argument, to the contrary, is that affect has never been separate from
reason. Affect is in fact enmeshed in reasoning, in that it 'point[s]
us in the proper direction, take[s] us to the appropriate place in a
decision-making space, where we may put the instruments of logic
to good use. ... Emotions and feeling, along with the covert physiological machinery underlying them, assist us with the daunting task
of predicting an uncertain future and planning our actions accordingly' (Damasio 2006: xxxiii).

Damasio proposes that the smart reasoning system evolved as an
extension of the automatic emotional system, with emotion and affect playing diverse roles in the reasoning process. This is because
the machinery by which we reason – what he refers to as the higher
brain – developed out of the machinery by which we feel (the lower
brain, where affect is 'felt' as a form of survival strategy). The older
communication system, which relied on chemical messengers in the
blood (hormones) was built on to create a more sophisticated sys-

tem that sent messages faster via neurons. The power of 'higher reasoning' ('mind'), created by this more sophisticated system, is not separate from the older system ('body') but intimately bound up with it. Sometimes affect, Damasio says, *can* substitute for reason: when we are fearful, for instance, it gets us out of danger before we verbalise or make conscious our reasons for doing so.[6] But reasoning gives us the chance to do this knowingly and an ability to act in determined ways.

So unlike women who claim that maternal instincts 'naturally' push one towards attachment parenting, it is not the case that we must act on this low-level reasoning; indeed, we have the power not to act in that particular way – and this is part of, as Descartes says, what makes us human. Nor is it the case, however, as Bobel suggests, that this 'low level reasoning' is a separate and irrelevant part of the higher-minded reasoning process. In our assessments of how to go about evaluating whether one is doing the 'right' thing, an attention to affect over reason need not denigrate any particular ethical principle: 'The fact that acting according to an ethical principle requires the participation of simple circuitry in the brain core does not cheapen the ethical principle. The edifice of ethics does not collapse, morality is not threatened, and in normal individuals the will remains the will' (Damasio 2006: xxiii–xxiv).

It would be undesirable to tie a defence of embodied knowledge to the language of science – rather, the intention is to show that reason and affect need not be mutually exclusive. Some scholars have even tried to integrate such an approach in their work on wider political schema. Connolly (1999), writing on secularism, makes an argument for attention to the affective life of political subjects. Again using a framework derived from neuroscientific studies, he argues for a two-tiered, but integrated, model of human reasoning. As he puts it, without both reason and affect, neither would intensity of feeling reach the higher brain, nor would we have the capacity for complex thought and judgement.

Rose's work has pointed out that in the age we live in, we are expected – encouraged even – to reflect upon and try to improve these 'pre-conscious' modes of intensity (Rose 1999), attempting to cultivate our capacity to listen more attentively to our inner selves to participate in a politics of becoming; a process particularly relevant to a focus on motherhood (Connolly 1999: 176). In fashioning our selves through these strategies, we are engaging in identity work, a project intimately tied up with our sensory experience.

Affect, Sensuality and Breastfeeding

In 'Weaning', Melanie Klein writes that 'only one part of ... satiation [in being breastfed] results from the alleviation of hunger ... another part, no less important, results from the pleasure which the baby experiences when his mouth is stimulated by sucking at his mother's breast' (Klein 1975: 290). Breastfeeding 'matters' because 'the first gratification which the child derives from the external world is the satisfaction experienced in being fed.... Analytic work has shown that babies of a few months of age certainly indulge in phantasy-building.... The object of all these phantasies is, to begin with, the breast of the mother (Klein 1936: 209, in Sutherland 1999: 4).

Throughout this book, there have been examples of women's identity work as they fashion themselves as (good) mothers through the prism of doing the 'best' thing for their child – as they see it, full-term, on-cue breastfeeding. One accountability strategy that sits well in a framework of intensive mothering is that which stresses how much the child *enjoys* the breastfeeding, and how devastated the child would be if it were stopped. One mother mentioned, in an interview about her attempts to wean her child, that her daughter's tears and tantrums when told that 'boobies would have to go bye-bye' were enough to 'break her heart':

> Virginia [*24, breastfeeding her 17-month-old daughter*]: I just couldn't do it, you know? There she was, absolutely inconsolable, doing these big gulping sobs, and I just thought, this is stupid. This is making me miserable, and her miserable. Why should I wean her just because people have a problem with it? She obviously still needs this [*pointing at her breasts*]. Once I realised that actually I *didn't* really want to wean her, I just got on with it – it stopped being a hardship and I just went with the flow.

Virginia makes the point that continuing to breastfeed feels right not only because it is what her child wants, but also because *she* enjoys it. Yet the extent of maternal enjoyment in breastfeeding is something that has long been considered problematic. Jane's comment hints at this crossover:

> Jane [*Leader applicant, 25, breastfeeding her 16-month-old son*]: ... you can't spoil a baby! Not with love and comfort. And sometimes, with [baby], He is always busy when he is awake so when I am breastfeeding him it is the only time he is looking into my eyes, and I can't describe it, you know, we are right there.... It's like we are in love or something. It's amazing, really.

Certainly, one of the most frequently proffered reactions to the subject of this study, from colleagues as much as friends, is that the women who breastfeed their infants into childhood must have 'something a bit Freudian going on' and the child will grow up to have 'issues'. And indeed, for Freud, any overlap between parenting and sexuality was pathological. Using anthropological studies of totemism, as well as his own self-analysis, Freud developed the Oedipus complex to explain how the self (specifically the superego) was formed. He argued that a male child's psychological development goes through the stage of selecting the mother as the object of libidinal investment – though the infant senses that this will anger the father, with a probable outcome of castration.[7] The infant internalises his father's rules, therefore creating the reflexive, superego. The father becomes the child's primary source of identification, as he wishes to keep his phallus. He stops attempting to have the mother, turning his attention to other objects of desire (Freud: 1977: 238). As Sutherland writes:

> Freudian theory centers on prohibitions against parental skin and touching; indeed, Freud worked to 'cure' patients who described sexual molestation, arguing that they had merely, in his determination, had particularly visceral Oedipal fantasies. The abstraction of flesh (especially sexualized flesh) to fantasy is essential to Freud's oedipal complex; indeed, the oedipal complex might be understood to represent a complex of separations – body from mind, adult from child, 'truth' from 'fantasy'. (Sutherland 1999: 5)

A common assumption is that the child has somehow been held back in infancy by the mother who continues to breastfeed him, perhaps as part of her own need to 'feel needed' by not allowing the child to separate from her (see also Chapter 3). The mother therefore remains the child's primary object of desire (and, arguably, he hers).

A large body of evidence undoubtedly 'point[s] to a definite connection for some women between breastfeeding as the transference or gifting of bodily nourishment and breastfeeding as a pleasurable sensory, possibly even erotic or sexual experience' (Shaw 2003: 63). Robinson is typical of comments I often heard when she says that this is 'completely normal' – again relying on hormones by way of explanation:

> During breastfeeding, two hormones are busy at work. Prolactin is producing milk, and oxytocin (the love hormone) is sending the message to bring down hindmilk. Some women have a distinct feel-

ing in their breasts, known as letting down, when this occurs. It can be experienced as a tingling sensation. The same hormones used in lovemaking are used in breastfeeding too. It's not unusual for some women to feel this sensation genitally as well. It's absolutely nothing to be ashamed of, or to feel uncomfortable about. It's normal. It's *completely* normal. (Robinson 2007: 21, emphasis in original)

Yet women are again in a bind here: breastfeeding promotion typically relies heavily on a discourse of breastfeeding being an asexual experience (although see Figure 2.1). Women themselves are left to find some way of negotiating this paradox. Judy does so by pointing to the 'mental and physical' difference between her husband's sexual attentions at her breast and those of her children, noting that they are 'completely different' sensations, which are not the same at all – because of how *she* understands them. Arguably, the sensation of one or other at the breast is the same 'affect,' but different 'emotion':

> *Judy [39, breastfeeding her 2- and 4-year-old daughters]*: And of course you have other people who see breasts just for sex ... if you want to talk about that? From my own personal experience, I mean, I do still have a sexual relationship with my husband, and I don't have as much energy as I would if I weren't breastfeeding, but, he, you know, this [gesturing a baby under her arm] is not what men do, you know, they can try, but they can never replicate. It is a completely different sensation, someone latching on, and someone having a play, which is not just mental but physical too. I don't know, I haven't had experience with breastfed men, but for me, it's just different.

For Blaffer Hrdy, who uses an evolutionary paradigm, 'maternity is inextricably intertwined with sexual sensations, and it is an infant's business, through grunts and coos, touches and smells to make the most of Mother Nature's reward system, which conditions a woman to make this infant a top priority. Evolutionary logic is firmly on the side of mothers who enjoy the sensual side of mothering for its own sake' (Blaffer Hrdy 2000: 538). In resolving the tension between sexuality and maternity, she takes an unconventional view on the subject:

> To classify maternal sensations as 'sexual' and therefore in puritanical minds to condemn them, is to privilege sexuality in a very non puritanical way, implying that sexual sensations are more important than equally powerful sensations that reward women for caring for babies. *We might just as logically describe various orgasmic contractions during love making as 'maternal'.* These responses by a lactating mother mammal to her baby's sucking long antedated sexual responsiveness to breast

stimulation in heterosexual (or any type of intimate) contacts. Propaganda from andocentric sources like *Playboy* notwithstanding, the feelings we identify as sexual were originally maternal. That is why, even in contemporary women, it should not surprise us that erotic arousal in the mother during breastfeeding can be correlated with increased milk ejection. (Blaffer Hrdy 2000: 537–538, emphasis in original)

Blaffer Hrdy contends there may be no contradiction in breastfeeding being both maternal and sexual. But she makes little comment on how this contradiction unfolds as the child ages. Is there a point at which it is too late in terms of the child's development, sexually or otherwise? If something 'feels right' but is considered, by law, to be dangerous or pathological, how does it serve as an accountability strategy? There have certainly been cases of the law considering a breastfeeding relationship between a mother and her growing child as sexually dubious and potentially abusive. Umansky (1998), for example, writes about the Karen Carter case in the United States, in which, after the mother told a counsellor she was worried about feeling sexually aroused when breastfeeding her 18-month-old child, the child was taken into care. La Leche League has supported women in these situations, validating mothering scenarios in which the status quo is disrupted by nursing beyond typical time frames.

The problem with a focus on affect at a policy level, of course, is that what 'feels' right to one person will not 'feel' right to another, as bodies are experienced differently by individuals, albeit in culturally pattered ways. My intention here has not been to suggest that this is an area policy makers should focus on, but rather to broaden the debates beyond 'informed choice' (see also Hausman on the need to go 'beyond science', 2003). Contrary to the policy focus, what these comments from mothers point to is that 'science' does not, and should not, dictate what people do.

Non-nutritive Sucking, or the Affective Residue

In the discussion of policy, law and pathology, the pleasurable and joyful side of the breastfeeding relationship that was so central for many of the women I spoke to, appears once again to have been eclipsed. Perhaps a 'residue' remains here that resists theorisation, or even verbalisation. If it does, it certainly does not sit easily within a legal framework.

Woodburn (2006), writing about her experience of breastfeeding her 4-year-old child, says simply that although she knows full well that her child did not 'need' breast milk in any nutritional sense, she continued to engage in what is termed 'non-nutritive sucking' (in effect, sucking for comfort, typically as part of a bedtime ritual). As she says, what does one do 'when physical nourishment is almost beside the point, and what we are talking about is mostly the emotional kind?' She concludes, recounting her son's emotional struggles with weaning:

> As a mother-to-be, I had carefully weighted the nutritional benefits of breastfeeding, but I hadn't considered this; a benefit as simple and powerful as a happy memory ... in this, as in many other parenting dilemmas, I've come to rest on hope as on fact, and more on our own idiosyncratic story than on any official one. Dostoevski wrote that a single happy memory might be all a man needs to avoid despair. My son will probably have many.... And maybe one day that will matter more than either of us can know right now (Woodburn 2006).

Whilst an accountability based on affect, like those based on nature or science, is full of contradictions, I wonder whether such a strategy might be productive, both in relation to breastfeeding and in other areas of personal life. In life, not everything one does can be explained and accounted for in the language of rationalism. In *Of Milk and Miracles*, Sutherland (1999) draws again on Klein to speak about her own experiences, using a framework of mutual attachment/detachment (taken up in the next chapter). She stresses the preverbal yet relational aspect of breastfeeding known only to the mother and child. Perhaps fittingly, then, someone else's experience is used to close this section of the discussion:

> Klein understands that it is not only the baby who needs to be filled, it is not only the baby's desires that matter; the mother needs to be filled with milk and desire too for, 'if she can enjoy [breastfeeding] thoroughly, her pleasure will be unconsciously realized by the child, and this reciprocal happiness will lead to a full emotional understanding between mother and child.' This is not a martyrdom or a sacrifice of one to the other, but a 'full emotional understanding between mother and child' ... [Drawing on her own experiences, she says] **You always want to stuff your fingers in my mouth while I nurse you; you want me to suck too ... You cannot speak yet, and I cannot speak with your fingers in my mouth, but we have things to teach each other, you and I, knowledge to share like a feast that has been divinely blessed. You smile at me dumbly, and I**

smile back, and we know what we mean' (Sutherland 1999: 18, emphasis in original).

Notes

1. One can also 'read' affect in nonverbal forms such as gestures, touches or looks. I have restricted my analysis largely to the problem of representation where verbal communication is limited, but appreciate that a more holistic approach may be warranted.

2. This might also explain why mothers who cannot breastfeed are frustrated and have feelings of failure. The distress of a screaming baby who cannot be pacified is at once the distress of the mother. Patricia, above, says one of the best things about breastfeeding is that she is able to soothe her child, 'a lifesaver emotionally for me'.

3. Discussed in 'Following Your Instincts, Part I' (2008). The author uses the example of wasps that have a 'Fixed Action Pattern'. When wasps return with prey to their nest, they normally abandon it at the entrance for a few moments whilst they inspect the lair. If researchers move the dead prey whilst the wasps are away, on return, the wasps endlessly repeat the inspection process, despite no intruders having had the chance to enter. Only when the prey is left in its original spot (by the wasp) do the inspections cease.

4. Much of the literature on the 'anthropology of birth' school is part of the canon of attachment parents, who advocate 'natural birth' in line with the practices described by anthropologists in societies elsewhere.

5. The authors stress that intuition is generally considered 'unscientific' and therefore devalued – yet intuition is increasingly defined in scientific terms as inherent to the basic structure of the nervous system (e.g., 'reason' being the product of left-brain thinking and 'intuition', right-brain). Advocates of 'intuitive knowledge' yet again frame their arguments in the language of science, never challenging this hegemony (Apple 2006; see Chapter 7).

6. At many of the conferences I went to during fieldwork, women were encouraged to tune in to their 'primal brains' to enable instinctive mothering, by being shown evolutionarily inspired slides of the primal brain. To some extent what I attempt to do here is reconcile this endeavour with space for reason and reflexivity in parenting, once again separating description (the 'is') from prescription (the 'ought').

7. He argued in later work that females also experience the Oedipus complex, initially directing (homosexual) desires towards the mother.

Part IV

Contextualising
Intensive Motherhood

Chapter 9

MOTHERING AS IDENTITY WORK
IN COMPARATIVE PERSPECTIVE
THE CASE OF FRANCE

Angela:[1] There is something incredible, something wonderful about breastfeeding. It goes on; it's like the fourth trimester ... breastfeeding manages to allow ... you to connect with the baby.

Having considered women's accountability strategies, the analysis turns back more strictly to the question of maternal subjectivity – specifically looking again at how relatedness is envisaged in conjunction with notions of the self. This chapter presents some accounts of this subjectivity from attachment mothers in London before turning to data from fieldwork in Paris. These data provide a contrast to the UK analysis, clarifying culture-specific issues around mothering and identity work. The argument is that the merged mother-infant self witnessed amongst the attachment mothers in the UK is an intensification of a more generalised intensive parenting culture, which encourages absorbed parenting on the part of mothers. The same mothering looks very different in a culture where mother-infant separation and autonomy is lauded as ideal, i.e., in the culture of non-intensive parenting currently found in France. Whereas women in the general LLL London group typically understood breastfeeding as a means of cultivating attachment, women in the general LLL group in Paris (that is, not 'attachment' mothers) use it as a means of mediating separation, reflecting broader cultural notions of subjectivity.

Making Selves: Separation and Attachment

A book that attachment mothers in London referred to frequently when speaking about mother-infant subjectivity was Kaplan's *One-*

ness and Separateness: From Infant to Individual (1978). A mix of psychoanalytic insights and parenting advice, the book opens by saying: 'In the first three years of life every human being undergoes yet a second birth, in which he is born as a psychological being possessing selfhood and a separate identity. The quality of self an infant achieves in those crucial three years will profoundly affect all of his subsequent existence' (Kaplan 1978: 15). A well-adjusted child, it is argued, should separate from its mother by degrees (i.e., via a philosophy of attachment parenting) rather than rushing through the stages of separation, as is more typical in wider society. Kaplan argues that individuation in the child (going from seeing oneself as an extension of the mother towards seeing oneself as an agential, separate entity) comes from an appreciation of 'the inner mother' imprinted in the child through early experiences of mothering. Not allowing this imprinting to happen can leave the child in a state of limbo between oneness and separateness: 'When this process goes wrong, a human being will have difficulties loving others, nurturing the young, taming his own aggression, knowing the boundaries of immediate time and space, mourning the dead and caring about the destiny of the human species' (Kaplan 1978: 19).

It was noted in Chapter 3 that the first fact of English kinship is the individuality of persons (Strathern 1992b). For Strathern, English people arrive attached, are 'separated' through socialisation, and thereby become able to 'relate' to others as individuals. Being able to (re)attach themselves autonomously to others allows them to participate in society. For the women in LLL groups in London, however, breastfeeding is a primary means by which to prolong the attachment of their children. They talked actively of the mother-infant dyad as needing 'protection' from a society that demanded separation. For them, separation need not be cultivated (or, at least, rushed), because being attached to the mother serves as a template for being attached to others (and, in due course, securing individuality). The same end is aspired to, but reached by different means.

The interesting question is why the attachment mothers, with their more magnified internalisation of this injunction, so strongly resist the separation they associate with 'normal' practices of the perinatal period, such as cutting the umbilical cord, formula feeding or separate sleeping. Borrowing an idea from Miller (1997), this language of individuation and attachment is, arguably, about creating not only the child's sense of self, but also that of the mother, which is embodied in a 'dual persona'.

Miller (1997) describes the 'semi-cultic' practices of the National Childbirth Trust groups he attended as rites de passage through which women negate their previous values and purify themselves in preparation to become new beings. He inverts traditional psycho-analytic theory from Klein to ask whether the stages a child is said to undergo (paranoid schizoid, depressive or otherwise) might not best be applied to the development of new mothers. Klein (1975), for example, argued that the paranoid-schizoid position occurs in infants when they cannot understand how the mother can be both the 'good breast' and the 'bad breast' – the source of all things good, and bad. Miller says the same is true for the mother, for whom the child is at once the source of all things good and all things awful. Breastfeeding is but one example of the child's perceived need being both enjoyable and constraining:

> The infant's constant demands are accepted as essential priorities and at no point should the mother's own desires prevent them being attended to.... All her skills of self-construction through agency become negated. This negation is acceptable because the baby is not viewed as another, but as part of the newly recycled dual persona of mother-infant. This may be related to Freud's observation that 'Parental love, which is so moving and at bottom so childish, is nothing but the parents' narcissism born again, which, transformed into object-love, unmistakably reveals its former nature.' (Freud 1984 [1914]: 85, in Miller 1997: 72–73)

Indeed, psychoanalytic literature has focused on the transformation of the mother during the process of birth and post-partum life. This is considered a time of psychic crisis that prompts her to work through her own infantile issues (Baraitser 2006). Typically, it is suggested that although a mother extends herself (literally, she reproduces), she also loses something. Naomi Wolf writes, for example: 'When I spoke to new mothers, it seemed to me that although a child and new love has been born, something else within them had passed away, and the experience was made harder because at some level, underneath their joy in their babies, these women were quietly mourning for this part of their earlier selves' (Wolf 2001: 6). The implication here is that a mother's self is changed irrevocably, demanding that a woman leave behind her previous, unified self and embrace a dyadic existence (however illusory the unified self might have been).

Generally, attachment mothers had a mixture of feelings on this issue. Amelia said, for example: 'Sometimes we have a great time and co-operate and other times I shout or feel dominated by my child'. Another mother mentioned various factors contributing to a sense of balance:

Questionnaire: Is it hard to balance your own needs with those of your child or children?

Claudine [24, breastfeeding her 17-month-old daughter]: Not really because I am not the self-sacrificing type at all! First, most of my needs do not exclude her or contradict hers, second I do always take the time to fill my own needs for as I say I am not the self-sacrificing type at all, and also she seems to understand my needs and gives me the space to fill them. But I guess this also because her dad is a great father, which allows me to have my own space. I suppose it might be more difficult with two or more children, or no daddy on hand.

A topic that came up frequently at meetings was the point at which a child's needs became wants, whereupon a child might be asked to wait to be breastfed, for example, or a mother might put her own 'need' to sleep through the night above her child's 'wanting' night-time feeding.[2] These tensions are not confined to attachment parents, of course, but stem from wider realities parents must negotiate. Veronika Robinson notes, about full-term breastfeeding in particular, however:

Veronika [37, 8-year-old daughter, breastfeeding her 7-year-old daughter]: … it depends on the age of the child. Around two or three they are emerging in the world, and starting to see themselves as separate from the mothers, and so as a mother you have to let them explore, and sort of let them push the boundary; other times you have to create that boundary, that is what parenting is about. … And so, yeah, I mean, child-led weaning doesn't mean that the child determines every time they are going to breastfeed … it is different to when you have a tiny baby. Their wants are their needs at that point. … It might be that you say 'we are not going to do it in the day' or 'in the night,' whatever the mother's thing is, and I don't think there is anything wrong with it … I think once they are moving around it's important to say that, you know, because you will have some children that will have you on the couch all day breastfeeding![3]

Miller's observations are largely confined to the early period of the child's life (typically, before 6 months of age). There comes a time, he says, when the child pushes the boundaries of the 'newly recycled dual persona', and 'intervention' is required – such as when the child needs to be told, for example, to wait to be breastfed. This is when the child starts being seen as an 'individual'.

Paris: A Comparison

The inflation (both ideological and material) of the dual persona that attachment parenting magnifies is a specific response to historical shifts in the UK, where emotionally absorbed parenting is lauded. This chapter now moves to an analysis of comparative ethnographic research carried out with members of La Leche League groups in Paris. Since women in France must return to work when their children are younger than their counterparts in the UK, pragmatic solutions for dealing with this separation (childcare, breast milk expression or formula feeding) are more prevalent. Parenting is less 'intensive,' and women are not engaging in self-realisation through parenting in ways described above. If anything, female strategies of identity work seem to be more concerned with questions of liberty and sexuality than mothering per se. Attachment mothers in France are therefore even more marginal than their UK counterparts. The focus is on women's experiences of negotiating an exacerbated 'cultural contradiction' while practising attachment parenting in Paris.

Why France?

Famously, the French government has long had a policy aimed at boosting the country's population, at the same time as increasing the number of women in the workforce (Randall 2000). The Organisation for Economic Co-operation and Development (OECD)[4] lists the fertility rate in France as 1.94, in contrast to the UK's 1.8. (These figures are both above the OECD average of 1.63).[5] In terms of female employment, 56.7 per cent of women of working age are employed in France, compared with 66.8 per cent in the UK. (The OECD average is 56.1 per cent, and this includes both full- and part-time workers).

At the time of research, in the UK a woman could typically expect 26 weeks (six months) of paid leave with five weeks additional unpaid leave if desired. (Women were not paid at full rate – it was calculated at 90 per cent for the initial six weeks and then at a flat rate, approximately 33 per cent of average wage, for 20 weeks).[6] In France, women could take 16 weeks of (fully) paid leave, then being eligible for longer periods of unpaid leave. Since this is generally split on a four-week/12-week basis pre- and post birth, women are expected to return to work when their children are between 10 weeks and 3 months old.[7] In the UK this point would typically be between 5 and 6 months. (Paternity leave at the time of research in both countries was two weeks, with only 25 per cent of this time paid in the UK).

Crucially however, and unlike the UK, France has a system of heavily subsidised, easily available, affordable childcare. Municipal, cooperative and parental crèches exist, able to care for infants from the age of 3 months at rates that are close to free through a system of pay-back from social security. From the age of 3 (or 2, in larger cities) children can attend pre-schools (*maternelles*) for eight hours a day, for free (with the option of a means-tested after-school and holiday club, available until 6.30 p.m.). By contrast, the average cost for a full-time nursery place for one child in London in 2005 was £197/week, or nearly £10,000/annum (Daycare Trust 2005). For French mothers, the need to 'juggle' careers around the demands of childcare following the end of maternity leave – practically and financially, at least – is mitigated.[8]

So whilst I do not expand on it here, these data clearly chime with, or are the flip-side of the coin to, those presented by scholars working on cross-cultural variations in welfare regimes (Esping-Anderson 1999, being the classic example). Where childcare is seen as the responsibility of the family it will clearly chafe with a dual-earner family set-up, therefore precipitating the full-time breadwinner/part-time carer model, with all its usual gendered implications. In France where the state takes more responsibility for care, it is understood as a means of protecting parents' (and particularly mothers') independence, economic and otherwise. Drawing on Pfau-Effinger's work, Edwards (2002) therefore makes the point that even for women who *do* work under the first model, such as the UK, child-care is understood as a mother-substitute, again resonating with the anxieties propagated by an intensive mothering ideology explored here, and particularly pertinent to the infant feeding question.

The French and British governments both advocate the WHO's recommendation that children should be breastfed exclusively for six months, and breastfed in conjunction with other foods for anything up to 2 years of age or beyond (WHO 2003). Initiation rates of breastfeeding stood at 78 per cent and 69 per cent in Britain and France respectively at the time of research,[9] with no formal statistics existing in either place for rates of breastfeeding at a year, or beyond. These numbers reflect the shorter length of maternity leave women receive in France, which in turn informs (and is informed by) broader social attitudes towards parenting and childcare.

Methodology

Four months of research were undertaken in Paris, following a pattern similar to that with LLL groups in London: I attended the monthly meetings of the six groups that operate within the Paris '75' region, as well as any family days, toddler meetings, LLL conferences or workshops. I also visited an LLL group in the suburbs of Paris to offer some comparison to these meetings.[10] In 2006 I attended the Grande Tétée, a large-scale public nurse-in in central Paris, organised by a group of mothers who all were also affiliated with LLL. Of particular interest in Paris were *réunions à theme*, organised by a group of attachment mothers connected largely through LLL, which explored in depth the philosophy of attachment parenting (*maternage proximal*) in meetings on the topics of breastfeeding and the life of the couple, non-violent discipline, breastfeeding whilst using a sling and so on. Rather like Attachment Parenting International meetings, these meetings served as forums for discussion of topics outside of the LLL breastfeeding remit. Meetings of the English-speaking LLL group in Paris, the original French LLL group, were also attended. This was a very active group made up of mothers from across the globe (largely American, German and English). Finally, I made visits to a local maternity hospital, the local milk bank and a lactation teaching hospital, as well as interviewing lactation specialists in the Paris region.

After attending the groups for some time, and having interviewed several mothers and LLL leaders in Paris, mothers at the groups were asked to fill out a questionnaire, a direct translation of that used in London. In Paris, one of the mothers in the first group I attended mentioned to me that she worked as a professional translator, and it was arranged that I would make a contribution to her LLL group (to allow her to participate at the national congress) in return for a translation that was sensitive to the LLL philosophy.[11]

The Context of Care

In France, private and public health-care systems operate in tandem. If one contributes to social security, one's family is entitled to subsidised or free medical and dental treatment. Maternity-related care is reimbursed at 100 per cent, midwife care at 70 per cent. Health treatments are assigned a basic monetary value, of which social security pays all or a proportion thereof. The remaining balance of bills (say, for midwife care) may be paid by a complementary health insurance scheme, to which many people subscribe.

As soon as pregnancy is officially confirmed, a woman is to inform her local Caisse d'Allocations Familiales, which will issue her *carnet de maternité*, to be presented to the hospital along with other documents required for hospitalisation. To qualify for social security maternity benefits, mothers must undergo four antenatal examinations during the third, sixth, eighth and ninth months of pregnancy, when scans are made to check foetal growth and detect abnormalities. Virtually all babies are born in hospital in France, with midwives handling most routine births and pregnancies. The percentage of women who give birth at home is very low in comparison with the UK (which itself is only around 2%), and it can be difficult to find a midwife willing to take on the responsibility of a home birth (Hampshire 2005).

Puericultrices in hospitals often look after babies and help women become familiar with the tasks of looking after a newborn. A stay of six days in hospital is typical (far longer than in the UK), and children are often left in nurseries overnight to allow mothers to rest: this was certainly the case at the maternity hospital in which I conducted fieldwork. Checks by paediatricians after the birth, and at eight days, are necessary for the *carnet de santé*. A mother must have a check-up at six weeks after birth. Whilst one can sign up for domicile service, in which a midwife comes to the home (like health visitors in the UK), in most areas postnatal checks are often done at mother and child protection centres, which provide free services to pregnant women and children under the age of 6. To be fully eligible for social service payments, further checks at 9 and 24 months are necessary.

Women in France receive five sessions of kinaesthetic treatment following the birth of their children to retrain their pelvic floor muscles. There is a strong emphasis on returning women to their pre-pregnancy figures as quickly as possible. One (British) mother told me her doctor in Paris had chastised her at her first postnatal appointment (five days after the birth of her son) for not having put on her make-up, and for having put on too much weight in pregnancy.

The women interviewed said doctors advised weaning children from the breast or bottle and onto solids at anything from 6 weeks to 3 months old. Although breastfeeding is technically encouraged, in reality little support or information about it is readily available from health professionals. The hospital where I conducted fieldwork had a room for the preparation of formula milk bottles, but no specialists to consult about breastfeeding. As discussed below, there are far fewer breastfeeding support organisations in France, and rarely are their members considered 'professionals' to the same extent as in the UK.

Doctor-patient relationships in France differ greatly from those in the UK, as a higher level of respect for the medical profession prevails in France. To a certain extent this is because the behaviour modification approach of the 'New Public Health' (Peterson and Lupton 1996) discussed in Chapter 2, so prevalent in the UK, is not typical in France. The idea of taking a birthing plan to the hospital in advance of the birth – which most mothers in my UK sample did, as patients 'enabled' to make such choices – was met with laughter by informants in Paris. One woman recounted how she had been told to look elsewhere if she disliked what the hospital would provide. French doctors were said to be more eager to preserve the traditional, paternalistic approach.

Not surprisingly, then, breastfeeding to full term goes against the grain of these institutionalised practices focused on establishing separation.[12] During research in France I was told about a child psychologist, Marchel Ruffo, who said that if he saw a 4-year-old breastfeeding, he would report it to the authorities (interview with long-standing LLL France leader).

LLL France

LLL France is not supported by any bursaries from the state, unlike LLLGB, which receives (or at least, has received) a grant from the Department of Health. This was a deliberate choice by the LLL France Council of Directors, which did not wish to be in a relationship of obligation with a state whose infant feeding policies and links with formula milk manufacturers it finds objectionable (interview with ex–Chair of Council). The French state has also been less forthcoming than the UK with funding for breastfeeding initiatives during the last twenty years. LLL France was founded in 1979, though meetings had been taking place amongst the anglophone group for some time before then. Part of the International Division of LLLI, it is within the Europe Area, unlike LLLGB, which as a separate affiliate of LLLI is less accountable to the central structure of the organisation and does not have to finance the activities of the Europe area from its own budget.

At the structural level, there are far more members per leader in France (ten) than in the UK (three). This is probably reflective of the fact that there are far more 'paid up' members of the group in France than in the UK (2,500 compared with about 900 in the UK), which is proportionally more per capita of the population. (LLL France National Congress, 2006).

A Divided Sample: The Context of Breastfeeding Support in France

The social contexts of breastfeeding support in France and the UK account for huge differences in the sorts of women who used LLL services, as reflected in the sample by two distinct groups: those who had come for a quick 'fix-it' solution for a breastfeeding problem, and those with a more specific interest in the philosophy of mothering through breastfeeding.

Many breastfeeding support organisations exist in Britain – perhaps because of the increasing attention paid to breastfeeding as a public health issue. In France it is not, as yet, a public health issue in the same way as in the UK. The UNICEF Baby Friendly Initiative has been very slowly taken up in France, and Paris had no accredited hospitals (there were only five in the whole country by 2007; the UK had fifty-one at the same point).[13] The post of lactation consultant, typically found in hospitals in the UK, is not recognised in France, and the government has only recently taken up the adoption of breastfeeding advocacy campaigns. Indeed, breastfeeding exclusively for six months, in line with the WHO guidelines, was recommended for the first time by the MS (Ministère de la Santé, Health Ministry) in its 2005 dossier, to great jubilation amongst informants here (though it should be noted that the MS had recommended breastfeeding in the past).

Yet breastfeeding is beginning to move towards centre stage in health policy, a fact reflected (and informed) by rising rates of initiation that increase each year – though this trend is largely reserved for the educated classes, as Amelie explains:

> Amelie [*32, breastfeeding her 2-month-old son, Questionnaire response*]: Breastfeeding has become very 'trendy' in the moneyed, well-educated classes, and I think that women choose it to be 'good mothers' … [Yet] I live in an area with a very high amount of recent immigrants to France, and for them, the bottle is better because it is synonymous with being moneyed ('the breast is for poor people').

La Leche League, as the only national breastfeeding support organisation,[14] therefore receives women from a diverse range of largely middle-class backgrounds (in the sense of being well educated), but certainly not only those with an interest in attachment parenting or long-term breastfeeding (as is more often the case in the UK). This, of course, causes some tensions within the group, as the purpose is to discuss the philosophy as much as aid women with a remedial 'fix-it' solution to their problems.

The 'fix-it' group formed the majority of my sample in France, whereas in the UK the reverse was the case. This was reflected in statistics showing that more women came to meetings when their babies were under 3 months old in France (nearly all of the mothers I met) than in the UK (about half), indicating an interest in breast-feeding largely within the brackets of maternity leave rather than for the 'long' term as attachment parents would prefer. This is probably a result of the rates of employment amongst women: whilst in the UK only one woman said that she was working full-time, and eight were working part-time (around a third), in France, seven (a third) were working full-time and five (a quarter) part-time. So, although overall the women were similar in several respects – married (around eight out of every ten couples), an average of 33 years old in France compared to 35 years old in the UK, and highly educated (with the vast majority in each sample having university-level qualifications) – the key difference was that in the French sample, many more women with young children were working outside of the home, reflecting the national policies described above (see Appendix 2).

This structural difference engendered different attitudes towards childcare, and particularly breastfeeding. In France, the average age of children being breastfed in the general group was 9 months, compared with 18 months in the UK – although this average probably obscures the fact that the French sample was divided largely between children being breastfed under 3 months (the fix-it group) and those with children over a year old (the attachment mother group). The average age of breastfed children in the attachment mother group in France (excluding those under a year old) was 17 months, compared with the 2¼ years in the UK, discussed above. The mothers questioned in the UK thought breastfeeding into the child's second year was ideal, whereas the average French respondent's ideal breastfeeding term was only up to one year (again, this average is skewed somewhat by combining women in two pronounced groups, whose answers alternated between 3 to 6 months and beyond a year).

Based on coding, just over a third of mothers answering the questionnaire in Paris (in both French- and English-speaking groups) met the attachment mother definition, compared with just over half in London. They constituted themselves as marginal in relation to French society at large, framing their answers to my questions with complaints about their own marginality in ways that, though more pronounced in France, were familiar from my experience in the UK.

Doubled Reflexivity

The anglophone LLL group was the first LLL group established in France. It held meetings as early as 1974, courtesy of a leader who had been trained in the US and then moved to Paris. Today it remains a thriving group for English-speaking women from all over the world. The women in my sample from this group came from Germany, the United States, Malaysia, the UK and India, and all were fluent in English. The narratives of these expat women are profiled here as a lever into a discussion of French parenting practices. Coming from foreigners in Paris who practised attachment parenting (as all in this case did), their comments are doubly reflexive about mainstream patterns of childcare. On the whole, these women viewed 'traditional' French childbirth and parenting practices very negatively, considering them overly medicalised, too focused on the mother's needs and not enough on the child's. Helga, a German woman, mentioned work as a factor:

> *Questionnaire*: Do you think that women are under pressure to feed their infants in a certain way at certain times?
>
> *Helga [38, breastfeeding her 6-month-old son]*: Yes
>
> *Questionnaire*: If yes; please say how so, and how this has influenced your own experiences:
>
> *Helga*: I have the impression that in France, many mothers are still talked into bottle-feeding, so that they can return to work when their child is three months old. It influenced me in the way that I looked for support already while being in the last trimester of my pregnancy.

Nayanika, a Malaysian-Indian woman in the group, commented on her French husband's approach:

> *Charlotte*: Was it something you had discussed with your husband beforehand [breastfeeding long-term]?
>
> *Nayanika [28, breastfeeding her 1-year-old daughter]*: No. [But] we did say we'd breastfeed.... My husband comes from a very traditional French family where babies are just left to scream their heads off and left to play alone for hours on end. Even though he's not like that and he sees the value in what we're doing I sometimes think he feels 'do we really need to be SO attentive?' It does cross his mind sometimes. When push comes to shove he would never leave her to cry. He's very attached to her. He sleeps next to her at night, and all that helps.

The isolation many of these women felt, as expats with few or no friends or family in close proximity, certainly seemed to breed a desire for group membership. The structure of the LLL organisation with its round of meetings gave women a framework to participate in and a network of friends to draw upon. This was particularly welcome to women who were not working outside the home (in all but one case, the women had arrived in Paris as a result of their partner's career).

Yet there are other groups in Paris for expat parents, most obviously Message, a large network of parents in the Paris region that organises parent- and child-related activities, though not with an exclusive focus on breastfeeding. So these women were also drawn to LLL for its specific philosophy, and it was interesting that the anglophone group was noticeably more interested in attachment parenting than the rest of the French LLL groups.

It is hard to suggest why this might be. It is true that in defining themselves against mainstream French methods of childcare, some members of this group considered themselves privy to better, more up-to-date information about appropriate care and frequently cited the work of American authors such as the Searses. There is a dearth of French-language texts on attachment parenting, and the only major author on the topic in French is a long-serving member of LLL France. Indeed, even LLL's *Womanly Art of Breastfeeding* has yet to appear in France in a fully serviceable translation; it is currently only available in a Canadian French version that contains useless references to local sources of support. (At the time of writing, one of my informants was working on a new translation.) Similarly, many women felt that as foreigners they had a licence to 'be different', an option they agreed was less possible for native women. Many of the women I spoke to relished this privilege – as Helga put it, 'I just think, you poor skinny French women! I'm so glad that being German gives me a licence to put on a bit of weight in pregnancy and not worry about getting my boobs out in public so much! God, who would want to be *French*?'

French Parenting: Non-intensive Motherhood?

Warner (2006), writing about her experience of motherhood in Paris, argues that unlike in her native US (and, I suggest, the UK), motherhood was far less intensive – it was not such a 'Big Deal' in France, and certainly not something women would consider their primary source of identity work. Indeed, for the most part there was far less fetishisation of the role of 'mother' among the women

I worked with in France – whereas 11 out of 25 UK women listed their 'profession' as 'Mum' in the questionnaire, only 1 in the sample of 19 women did so in France. Women were generally less effusive about the 'wonders' of motherhood in their answers to the questionnaire (unless they were in the attachment group). For example, they often answered the question 'Why was it important for you to feed your child at the breast?' in a single word, in contrast to long essays from UK mothers or attachment parents in France.

In the French LLL groups, fewer women said they felt a need to 'explain their decisions about how they feed their infants to other people', a third replying 'yes' compared with half the mothers in the UK sample, suggesting the latter had a heightened awareness of their own accountability or reflexivity – about this, at least. The argument is that in France, there is less plurality regarding infant care: mothers in general must go back to work earlier, which limits their ability to, for example, breastfeed to full term; consequently less identity work is required about one's decisions, in the form of accountability. By the same logic, those who do breastfeed to full term in France require even more identity work than their UK counterparts.

It seems that in France, there is not (yet) an industry surrounding parenting like the one in the UK. A search for 'parenting' on the Google UK site generates 85,100,000 results; a search for '*parentage*' in Google France yields just 1,660,000.[15] The style of politics discussed in Chapter 1 is less prevalent in France, and 'parenting' has not become a policy buzzword. As the American author Warner explains, this lack of 'support' for parents is double-edged, because while it collapses choice, it also reduces anxiety and accountability. As she writes of her experiences:

> Guilt just wasn't in the air. It wasn't considered a natural consequence of working motherhood.... The general French conviction that one should live a 'balanced' life was especially true for mothers – particularly, I would say, for stay-at-home mothers, who were otherwise considered at risk of falling into excessive child-centeredness. And that, the French believed, was wrong. Obsessive. Inappropriate. Just plain weird. (Warner 2006: 10–11)

Regarding her work in France, Wolfenstein (1955, with Margaret Mead) noted that for the Parisian parents she studied in the 1950s, childhood was not about fun but about *preparation*. This was, she argues, in almost direct contrast to her native United States, where 'childhood is a very nearly ideal time, a time for enjoyment, an end in itself' – in France, 'childhood is a period of probation, when everything is a means to an end; it is unenviable from the vantage point of adulthood' (Wolfenstein 1955: 115). In contrast to my informants in the UK who practised mothering as identity work, adults in France do not expect children to disrupt adult life, and children should certainly not be the main preoccupation of adult conversation, for example (Wolfenstein 1955: 114). The idea that activities should be child-centred, or that the smallest influences in childhood can massively affect adult outcomes, is not prevalent to the same extent. Children are not considered vulnerable, nor parents omnipotent, and in need of 'support.' Mother-blame and mother-guilt are not (yet) institutionalised.

This is reiterated in more recent research by Suizzo, published in *Ethos* (2004). In her article 'Mother-Child Relationships in France', she used a cultural models framework to argue for two distinctive features of French parenting. One was that mothers wanted their children to be '*Debrouillard*', a difficult term to translate into English that broadly means being prepared and therefore enabled to manage for oneself and achieve one's personal goals. The second, more pertinent feature was a pervasive worry about mothers being enslaved to their children (*esclavage*), who could easily become infant kings (*l'enfant-roi*). As Suizzo explains: '[Esclavage] is the idea that mothers can become dependent on, even subordinate to, their children. This notion is quite different from the much more pervasive concern among parents in individualist cultures that children may become overly dependent on their mother. Mother-enslavement was described as a loss of personal freedom with very negative consequences for the mother' (Suizzo 2004: 317).

Note that Suizzo says it is the mother who is suspect here. The fear of enslavement means that French parents 'prefer more distal relations, maintaining separate beds and bedrooms for their infants, and engaging in less body contact, in part because they believe that separateness fosters independence in children … French parents also avoid prolonged body contact, such as co-sleeping, holding, and carrying babies. … These findings point to a concern with fostering independence' (Suizzo 2004: 296). Weaning would be a good example of a practice ensuring that distal relations are maintained. As a social transformation that is not socially marked through ritual, the elasticity of the process presents a challenge for the mother. Breastfeeding is the means by which she mediates this separation, as Louise, a member of LLL France, makes evident:

Charlotte: Can you tell me what breastfeeding represents, to you?

Louise [28, just weaned her 6-month-old daughter]: It was the 'fusioned' aspect most of all, between mother and baby. Privileging all of the senses; touch, smell. In fact, I had a lot of trouble separating myself. So after 6 months it was a good moment to stop being so close to her.

There is an implication here that although breastfeeding is enjoyable for both the mother and the child, being 'close' for too long is undesirable. Suizzo argues that these ideas come from Rousseau, who wrote:

The first tears of children are prayers. If one is not careful, they soon become orders. Children begin by getting themselves assisted; they end by getting themselves served. Thus, from their own weakness, which is in the first place the source of the feeling of their dependence, is subsequently born the idea of empire and domination. (Rousseau 1979: 66, in Suizzo 2004: 317)[16]

One mother practising attachment parenting echoed the view that the French were concerned about women becoming '*mères fusionelles*':

Sandrine [28, 5- and 2½-year-old sons, no longer breastfed]: There is a massive misunderstanding around babies who breastfeed often, and for a long time … it is also difficult to breastfeed for longer than 4 to 6 months without being seen as a 'mère fusionelle' who is not able to separate from her baby.

Interestingly, she says that in France one would be considered suspect if one continued to breastfeed past 4 to 6 months – in the UK, this point would arguably be later, again reminding us of the symbiotic relationship between structural realities (maternity leave) and cultural values (when one is considered suspect).

It's Natural? Feminism and
(Full-Term) Breastfeeding in France

To understand why patterns of parenting – along with validations of personal liberty and emotionally absorbing parenting – are more or less salient in London or Paris, a broader cultural perspective is required.

The suggestion here is that in France, the attitude towards the place of nature is more 'embedded', in opposition to the growing fetishisation of nature as something desirable to 'get back in touch with' currently prevalent in the UK. True, Rousseau counselled women to 'look to the animals' in his campaign against wet-nursing in eighteenth-century France (Badinter 1981; Blaffer Hrdy 2000). But it would be fair to argue that over the last two centuries this injunction has faced rebuke from the legacy of the Enlightenment, which stresses human separation from nature and, in turn, other animals. Nicole put it in terms of culture:

> *Charlotte*: You said that in France there is not a 'breastfeeding culture' – why?
>
> *Nicole* [*Chair of Council*]: I think that in England there was always, at least for the last century and a half, a culture of returning to nature, proximity with nature, with one's choices, with people – there is a conscience about children that is much more ancient. In France, there was, by contrast, a 'hygienist' culture, with a very strict order, 'puéri-culture' centres, which set the rules: 'One must do it like this, and like that.' It's something that's very evident in the puéri-culture world today. It really harmed breastfeeding, and it's an approach that has never really been discredited. It just didn't fit with breastfeeding, where you can't be 'controlled by the rod', in such a rigid way.

The 'return to nature' in the 1970s that saw LLL blossom in the UK was not replicated in France – indeed, 'being close to nature' as something desirable is a relatively new phenomenon in France – a 'culture on the make' for a privileged section of society. This was even evident in the sorts of food mothers brought along to meetings. Whilst organic bread, cheese and vegetables were typical in the UK, in France it was normal to see packaged and processed foods – though there is a growing market for 'organic' (*biologique*) food in France, which may well start to feature in much the same way as in the UK.

When asked whether they considered themselves *alternatif* (alternative), women in the French LLL group typically did not understand my question, whereas in the UK the word was taken to be a label for a particular lifestyle that rejects certain 'mainstream' patterns. Yet the attachment mothers in France wholeheartedly agreed with the label and shared the views of women in the UK – lamenting that today what is 'alternative' is 'the most natural':

> *Questionnaire*: Do you consider yourself 'alternative'?
>
> *Daniele* [*30, breastfeeding her 16-month-old son*]: Yes, in motherhood in general, and it was already the case in other domains. It's funny to see that the most natural is 'alternative' these days!

As in the UK, attachment mothers in the French groups considered themselves 'beacons' who were 'spreading the light' about attachment parenting, in distinction to mainstream patterns of care.
Typically, and to a greater extent than in the UK, they spoke of their
marginalisation. Many women in this subsample said the reason
they enjoyed breastfeeding was that it was 'the closest to nature' – a
theme that cropped up increasingly in the promotion of breastfeeding. Yet for many women in the general French LLL group, the idea
of being 'a mammal' was both a reason to breastfeed and a reason
people were put off by it:

> *Sophie [25, breastfeeding her 3-month-old daughter, Questionnaire response]*:
> Breastfeeding seems like an animal act, uncivilised.

> *Simone [28, breastfeeding her 4-year-old son and 1-year-old daughter, Ques-
> tionnaire response]*: You probably know the documentary 'Baby of the
> World' [featuring images of older children being breastfed in other
> cultures]: When one sees that, one sees everything! Only, not in
> France, where we don't do like everyone else does. ... By contrast, I
> think that there are certain things that one can never change: we are
> mammals and that's that! Yes, sure, babies can survive with formula
> milk, because there are the medicines around that let them do that,
> but if we were elsewhere, it wouldn't work like that. So yes, I am
> alternative in France, and unfortunately I am obliged to realise that.
> But in a global sense, I'm not [alternative].

This ambivalence about our status as mammals was considered part
of the country's history of both the Enlightenment and feminism
– in contrast to the UK and US, where this discourse is frequently
drawn upon as a way of encouraging women to breastfeed. Accordingly, my French data draw me back to a discussion of feminism,
which yet again serves as a parameter of identity work. These different parameters reveal cultural norms surrounding femininity and
motherhood.

> *Charlotte*: There is also the fact that one thinks of breastfeeding as
> 'esclavage'...

> *Nicole [Chair of Council]*: Yes, I agree, feminism was constructed out-
> side of and AGAINST motherhood. The battle of feminism was: equal
> salaries between men and women, for abortion to defend the sexual
> liberty of women ... but not at all in favour of motherhood, absolutely
> not! Whereas in other countries, such as Scandinavia, feminism was
> constructed WITH motherhood. Moreover, the majority of French
> feminists didn't have children ... like it was a liberty not to have chil-
> dren. Revenge against nature, yes, that's it, a controlling of nature.

To be free was to get out of that condition. It stopped there. The blow was that breastfeeding was seen as the 'esclavage' [slavery] of women ... [actually a very] chauvinist image of women who were reduced to their sole sexual function of making babies. This idea is still spread in the collective unconsciousness. Nowadays, it's false, since the most educated women breastfeed the longest, and they are reversing that image.

Speaking about a friend who did not breastfeed her child, Louise explained again that her reasoning was a product of French feminist thought, which does not encourage women to adjust to the 'rhythm' of their children, but vice versa:

Charlotte: Why do you think your friend didn't want to breastfeed?

Louise [28, just weaned her 6-month-old daughter]: In '68 there was a big revolution, the liberation of women and all that ... so in our parents' generation there weren't many feminists who breastfed. And even now there is an image of the modern woman: she has five arms and six legs, she goes everywhere, does everything, she works and she is not dependent on anyone and above all not to her children. When one breastfeeds, one has another rhythm, one is obliged to adapt to the rhythm of the child...the child has become a 'child-king', but the mother is woman before being mother.

Charlotte: It's interesting, the distinction between motherhood and womanhood...

Louise: When one looks at northern societies [such as Scandinavia], it's different, women don't get posed the same question [to breastfeed or not]: they breastfeed. If they do not breastfeed they are not considered good mothers. Whereas in France, it's the opposite, it's the woman who breastfeeds who is thought of badly, and who is thought 'strange'.... One must go back to work early ... I took holiday, and after, I had holiday to use up ... like that I was able to [breastfeed] for five months. In short, one has to fight to be able to breastfeed, one has to find combinations that work.

Thus many women were conscious that according to these cultural norms about bodies and dependency, using either formula or expressed milk made sense for mothers in France:

Diane [32, breastfeeding her 5-month-old daughter, Questionnaire response]: It can appear more practical to bottle-feed [with expressed milk] as one can better manage the rhythm of the feeds; the woman is not strictly tied to her baby (for me, the idea of expressing milk with a pump is pretty distasteful, so I sometimes time where I will be with breastfeeding, not wanting to or not able to take the baby out everywhere – cinemas and theatres, etc). The body of a woman who breastfeeds becomes totally maternal, and that can change the relationship one has with one's partner (especially if the breastfeeding is long-term).

In France, feminism was associated with the work of Simone de Beauvoir, particularly her 'existential feminism'. Her work *The Second Sex* describes how female physiology renders women subservient to the requirement that the species procreate, in ways vastly more costly than those accrued to men. She viewed breastfeeding as a sort of enslavement. As Aengst and Layne note, 'she celebrates human society which exerts mastery over nature: "[h]uman society is an antiphysis – in a sense it is against nature; it does not passively submit to the presence of nature but rather takes over the control of nature on its own behalf" (1989: 53)' (Aengst and Layne 2010: 73). Hence, breastfeeding at all is seen to be against the ethic of 'French' feminism. Breastfeeding 'to full term' makes one even more marginal.

There are, of course, counter-currents to this. An article appearing in *Elle* magazine, entitled 'The End of Feminism? What Happens When Super-Woman Returns to the House', featured two of my informants, describing their feminism in a language reminiscent of attachment mothers in London (Elle 2008):

> I never "found" myself in feminism. There are fundamental differences between men and women. Motherhood is an essential one. I intend to be a mother as much as a woman. I have the chance to work at home, so my son, who is nearly 3 years old, has never been looked after [by anyone else]. There is a rhythm with the rest of the world. I breastfed him for a long time, and until the age of 1 he was always by my side, in a scarf next to me. Yet, I have an active life; I am a journalist and a translator and I work in public associations. But to work should not be synonymous with separation from one's child. I do not want to impose that on him. Moreover, I did not register him at school: I like the idea of him being free in his activities.

Stephanie has managed to combine work with attachment to her child, but this is particularly difficult in France, where women are expected to be at work at a much earlier point. Those wanting to practise 'attachment' styles of care find themselves in an exacerbated cultural contradiction, especially where to be a feminist is to speak in the language of liberty:

> *Questionnaire*: Do you find it hard to balance your own needs with those of your child(ren)?

Maud [*35, breastfeeding her 6-month-old daughter*]: Yes, I have to admit, I don't have the time to look after my own needs, but this isn't my daughter's fault, nor that of the breastfeeding, but society which imposes a frenetic and stressful rhythm of life where motherhood such as it used to be is increasingly difficult: maternity leave which is too short, individualism and dispersion of families, 'equality' between men and women (which in practice means that women work like men – except for less pay! – and continue to take on the role of mother and housewife, that's to say, double work!... all as a result of wanting to be equal – 'hello victory!!)

'Réunions à thème': Attachment Mothers in Paris

Like attachment mothers elsewhere, women practising attachment parenting in France extend the period of the mother-infant dyad. Their general approach to parenting, which relies heavily on a validation of nature as opposed to culture, is not, in general, endorsed in broader French culture, which validates the Enlightenment legacy of humanism and domination over nature. They are therefore not seen to be helping a feminist cause – quite the reverse. Indeed, in her new book *Le Conflit: La Femme et la Mere*, the French feminist Elisabeth Badinter (2010) argues that French feminism is under threat from this new wave of 'eco-motherhood'. Breastfeeding for six months (not considered unusual within the realms of attachment parenting in the UK) would be considered radical in France, which has a stronger discourse of female liberty, not only from a woman's role as mother but as an autonomous person able to participate in the public sphere on equal footing with men.[17] Even for mothers who do choose to stay at home (and opt out of paid employment), as Warner argues, it is considered important to maintain a 'sense of self' by using childcare on a regular basis for fear of becoming too tied to one's children.

I noticed that women who did practise attachment parenting in France showed even stronger commitment to the cause than those in the UK, perhaps as a result of this exacerbated non-conventionality. They were not only involved in public campaigns to raise awareness of breastfeeding, but would hold special *réunions à thème* in Paris to discuss AP philosophy more fully, which is not strictly allowed under the LLL remit. Their email notes:

[14] The 'réunions à thèmes' are run by leaders from LLL, and a small group of active mothers [names] who are members of LLL groups

in the Paris region. We want to offer – to mothers in LLL groups in Paris and to other mothers/fathers interested in 'maternage proximal' – a chance to open up discussion on specific themes supporting mothering through breastfeeding: breastfeeding whilst using a sling, co-sleeping, non-violent education, etc. The speakers will be either LLL leaders or active mothers experienced in a particular subject. All volunteers, (speakers, hostesses, organisers), these meetings share the fruit of engagement, in the spirit of mother-to-mother support.

The *réunions à thème* brought together 'attachment mothers' from the French-speaking groups as well as many members of the English-speaking groups in Paris. One French mother, Maud, lamented that their practices were considered 'extreme' in France:

Maud [35, breastfeeding her 6-month-old daughter]: LLL has a double image: that of an association to support breastfeeding through [the provision of] information, and also an extreme image. We are in a society where one must respect the norms of early childhood, and the values of 'maternage proximal', the co-sleeping, the long-term breastfeeding, tandem nursing ... are often seen as extreme practices.

Another French mother, living in London, similarly noted:

Audrey [35, breastfeeding her newborn son]: My friends in Paris think I am totally mad for not wanting an epidural during the birth, and for breastfeeding for five months – if only they knew I might do it for five years! They say to me that I pick him up too much when he cries and that 'il faut frustrer le bébé' – I don't know how you would translate that, but it basically means I am making a rod for my own back by making a clingy baby, or 'you must frustrate the baby'.

Expressing Milk: The French Way?

So how do women negotiate competing discourses that stress feminine liberty yet are increasingly starting to advocate breastfeeding? In France, since many women return to work when their baby is only 10 weeks old, there was a greater demand for information about expressing milk than in the UK. Thus there were many more conversations about the best sort of breast pump and the storage of breast milk, as well as questions about how to get the baby to sleep through the night, and to eat solids, from as early as 3 months.

The expression of breast milk (by hand or with a pump, for feeding from a cup or bottle) has been central to the infant feeding issue in the US for some time, where six weeks of maternity leave is standard (Blum 1999). The practice is sold as offering the ultimate solution for working women, in part through the merging of the domestic and public spheres. Separating the product from the means of production means that the child benefits by receiving breast milk even when it is unable to extract it itself, or when the mother is absent. The mother is therefore able to invest her energies in other labours (such as employment). A woman doesn't have to expose her breast in public, a third party can engage in the feeding process (meaning that 'bonding' can be shared) and parents can see exactly how much the child is eating.

Yet critics of the 'pump-culture' claim that children (and mothers) miss out greatly by not actually being in skin-to-skin contact for feeding, and that feeding expressed milk to infants hinders jaw and eye development, puts the supply-demand relationship of milk production out of kilter, and disrupts the production of antibodies specific to the maternal-infant environment. Many breastfeeding advocates see any sort of separation, in the form of a bottle or teat, as damaging for the child. Some of the 'attachment mothers' were concerned that something essential to the mothering relationship – the bonding – was missing, when the contact between mother and baby was mediated by a bottle or pump.[18]

Many LLL leaders therefore understood expressing as less than ideal, meanwhile taking a pragmatic approach to women's general inability to delay their return to work in France. Whilst in the UK women were sometimes asked, by other LLL members or leaders, 'Could you possibly afford not to work?' this was rarely asked in France – tips on combining breastfeeding and working would be proffered instead.

Furthermore, although French women generally considered themselves to be less prudish about nudity than their British counterparts, they found the contradiction between 'le corps « maternel » et le corps « érotique »' more problematic than the majority of my British respondents, and there was an interesting difference in how British and French women narrated this contradiction: French informants seemed to prioritise descriptions of their bodies in their accounts of breastfeeding. For example, where women in France would talk about 'my breasts', women in Britain spoke of 'the breast'. Bobel notes that this latter term is a form of objectification that at once resists and accepts cultural prescriptions about breasts, put to the service of another (Bobel 2001: 136) – though I also remember one woman in the French maternity hospital who, when asked why she had chosen to formula feed, answered, 'My breasts are for my husband.'

'The body' has been the focus of much discussion in the social sciences, particularly since the arrival of technologies of modification. It is notable that breasts – in both the UK and France – are probably the greatest site of female bodily modification in the form of plastic surgery (which often precludes breastfeeding). In contradistinction to the typical emphasis in social science on the commodification and objectification of bodies, McDonald and Lambert, in their recent volume *Social Bodies,* aim to consider the extent to which 'bodies and their elements are themselves 'social'' (McDonald and Lambert 2009: 2). To this extent, breasts can be regarded as a site of women's identity work – albeit with different emphases in Britain and France, with respect to the transition between the maternal and erotic bodies. McDonald and Lambert note that the transformation of bodies is 'never confined solely to the biologically functional in their effects but inevitably entail[s] the reformulation, reconstruction or re-establishment of social relations between persons and between human groups' (2009: 5). We might say that the moral relations of accountability (to the child, or to the partner) are made corporeal by women through their breasts.

Thus, when women in the UK group mentioned co-sleeping as affecting their relationship with their husband, it would usually be in a dismissive tone. Generally, less 'intimacy time' with a partner was considered a reasonable sacrifice for a 'family bed' philosophy:

> *Judy [39, breastfeeding her 2- and 4-year-old daughters, Questionnaire response]*: Yes, our children have access to our bed and we do not exclude them from our evening time. Overall – bar a few bad colds and a few restless nights – we sleep very well, and are a very close family. I see it as a reflection of the commitment we have to the wellbeing of our girls and believe it has strengthened the relationship I have with my husband. The extra evening time our children have had, especially with their father, has been very important.

By contrast, Nayanika, in the Parisian anglophone group, told this story about her relationship with her (French) husband and her breastfeeding daughter:

> *Nayanika [28, breastfeeding her 1-year-old daughter]:* My husband was having his breakfast, and she started fussing. I was in the middle of making coffee and I just undid my bra. Then he said, 'I suppose that's why a lot of women don't breastfeed, because men stop feeling sexual afterwards. I've just grown to accept that they're [her breasts]

not mine anymore.' I don't feel sexual about my breasts any more as they're so nutritive and practical. It's not the same as before.

Most French LLL members I spoke with seemed more concerned about effects like these, speaking less about children's 'bonding' with the father than about the effect of their parenting practices on their intimacy as a couple:

> *Diane [35, breastfeeding her 3-month-old daughter, Questionnaire response]:* Effectively, to be able to breastfeed during the night, I moved her into our bed, which had a positive side, for being able to nurse whilst sleeping but also had negative effects:
>
>> 1. She wakes up more often, three times a night, whereas when she slept alone in her cradle she wouldn't wake up more than twice – I am more tired because my sleep is broken.
>>
>> 2. The intimacy with my partner has been really limited, and I think that to put her back into her own bed would be nearly impossible (But at the same time I wonder how and when? When will she sleep through?)

There is certainly a difference in the ease with which French women consider themselves able to 'sell' attachment parenting to their partners, when compared with their British counterparts. I cite the following conversation between myself and two members of the anglophone group in Paris to show how women negotiate these multiple accountabilities – in this case to their French husbands (who would prefer their wives to socialise more), and to their children (who, cared for according to attachment parenting guidelines, prevent them from doing so):

> *Charlotte:* Do you work?

> *Vicky [34, breastfeeding her 1-year-old daughter]:* I did, but … I want to stay with her as much as I can and I want to have another baby as well. I like the idea of having more kids.

> *Nayanika [28, breastfeeding her 1-year-old daughter]:* I like the idea as well – but three years of breastfeeding, times [multiplied by] however many children. I'm not sure my husband can take it! My husband definitely wants to stop at two. He loves it but I don't think he can do this life of staying-in. You have to stay in all the time. She won't go to bed with anyone but me.

> *Vicky:* Life is so different when you breastfeed this way. I see other mums who stopped breastfeeding much earlier and they go out to dinner once a week with their husbands. Their life is almost back to pre-baby social.

Nayanika: But I didn't have a baby to get back to pre-baby as quickly as possible. That's my logic. That's not entirely my husband's logic and I have to respect the fact that there are two people in this marriage and family. It's fair enough. I really wanted to get pregnant and he was less ready to have a baby.

Vicky: I often hear talking about people putting their baby to bed early, getting them to sleep from an early hour. But I don't want my evening back. I put her to bed early for her, but I would rather have her up with my husband and I. Though of course, I am tired.

Nayanika: I don't want to go and sit in a restaurant when I can be with her. [The time] is so precious and it goes by so quickly.

Vicky: I don't have the desire to go and sit in a restaurant.

Nayanika: I think from my husband it comes from the people around him. The fact that a lot of people have found having children so difficult. We really are freaks [compared to how the rest of our friends do it].

Vicky: I have other people who I'm in touch with who are like us, but we don't see our friends very often. We don't have people over for dinner, the husbands don't see each other any more. He's very different from his friends that he talks to, and to the people at work.

Charlotte: Not going out for dinner, and not meeting friends for a drink, I think that's something I would miss…

Nayanika: I do miss it, but only from a social perspective. Rather than go out, we have had people over for dinner but it's a circus. My husband ends up entertaining them a lot more than I do, and I go and put her to sleep which takes an hour.

Vicky: If I had my friends over for dinner, it would be [my husband] entertaining our friends and I would be in the bedroom with her.

Nayanika: It has spoilt some of my friendships. I know that [my daughter's] godmother is slightly disappointed that I've stopped working and I'm staying at home. She has a really high-flying job. She's surprised at me, and I see a lot less of her. She's found this whole side to me that she can't quite deal with. On the other hand I have some friends with whom I've got in touch with again, and some who think what I'm doing is really wonderful – and all the new people at LLL.

Conclusion

An interesting part of this discussion is how the experiences of French and British women who practise attachment parenting challenge the prevailing norms in each country. We see that the length of maternity leave routinely given to women, the importance of work outside of the home for self-realisation and notions of individual autonomy combine to have a substantial impact on how women go about narrating their experiences of parenting. Where in the UK, attachment parenting might be described as an intensification of the prevailing climate of 'intensive parenting' (prevailing for the middle classes, at least), in France, attachment parenting goes against the grain.

What this discussion does not highlight is the struggle of French women who would like to spend more time with their children in the early months and resent the social pressure to return to work, 'get their bodies back' or return to a 'pre-baby social life'. This struggle, however, emerges as a result of shifting cultural orthodoxies, which recently have seen a gradual turn towards intensive mothering, potentially making a language of 'guilt' long familiar to mothers in the UK all the more salient. How each group of women negotiates these shifts – one provided with an generous system of childcare, the other with a longer provision of maternity leave – will undoubtedly be a source of feminist interest for some time to come. As Badinter says:

> The majority of French women reconcile maternity with professional life. Many of them work full-time when they have a child. They are resisting the model of the perfect mother, but for how long? (Guardian 2010)

Notes

1. Member of the Breastfeeding Manifesto coalition, speaking in an interview.
2. The point at which a child is reflexive enough to have a 'want' rather than a 'need' is a matter of debate, as is the extent to which this is influenced by the mother's cultivation of his or her 'wants'. This paradox is reflected in much of the 'healthy eating' literature, which on the one hand stresses that babies and toddlers should be allowed to determine the length and frequency of breastfeeding, and on the other asserts that parents should provide children with 'healthy options' during the weaning process. Presumably, if toddlers were allowed to decide what they wanted to eat, this might contradict healthy eating advice. Again, this raises questions of autonomy and informed consent, the parameters of which are managed by mothers.
3. This is heavily affected by the different characteristics of each individual child:

Charlotte: Are there any downsides to long-term breastfeeding?
Leticia [*36, 3½-year-old son, breastfeeding her 2-year-old daughter*]: The things people say ... there is the element of being in demand all the time, of being attached to the baby all the time, and you can get around that with expressing, which I did, with my son ... but with my daughter, I haven't felt a need to do it, so I have felt quite happy to be attached to her. Maybe that is to do with her being an independent baby ... she is quite happy to be put down and crawl around and do her own thing, so I don't feel like I am carrying her the whole time, like a weight.

4. An organisation committed to democracy and the market economy, the OECD is based in France and has thirty member countries, including France, Germany, Italy, Japan, New Zealand, Australia, the UK and the United States,.

5. The following statistics are taken from the data set http://stats.oecd .org/wbos/default.aspx?DatasetCode=LFS_D (retrieved 2 December 2008).

6. This was the case at the time of research; recent (2008) measures have extended standard maternity leave to one year (Directgov 2011).

7. These were the national, standardised rates of maternity leave. Some women – particularly in the UK sample – had more generous maternity packages. Women also had the option of taking extended periods of unpaid leave.

8. Hays (1996) noted that 'intensive mothering' came about in the United States at a time when women were increasingly entering the workforce, precipitating the language of 'juggling'. It is interesting that this language is less prevalent in France, perhaps due to the different histories of feminism, discussed below.

9. These statistics should be read cautiously. 'Initiation' means that the baby is put to the breast once. By one week in the UK, over a third of women are not breastfeeding, and by six weeks, that figure is well over half (DH 2005d). At the time of research these were the correct rates from the DH and French Health Ministry surveys (MS 2005). The most recent *report* available in France (MS 2005), however, puts the rate of initiation at 52 per cent: with an average duration of ten weeks.

10. Paris is a far smaller region than London (with a population of 2,175,000 compared to 6,377,000 in London, which includes Greater London). In London, only one group operated in Central London (a region comparable to Paris proper). Thus I worked with groups in the Greater London suburbs, those reachable on London transport. In Paris, six groups operated within Paris proper, and several more outside (one of which I visited).

11. My own language skills are competent, but I felt happier having a professional translation in this case.

12. To take Strathern's argument, French kinship might be characterised by

an even stronger emphasis on the need to separate before being considered a social actor.

13. Retrieved 23 April 2009 from http://www.lllfrance.org/allaitement-information/hopital-ami-bebe.htm#

14. With the exception of Solidarilait, which is more strictly a campaigning organisation.

15. Indeed, the word 'parenting' as a description of a genre of literature is under debate, which is an interesting social comment in itself. In place of *Parentage*, some informants would use *Parentalité* (parenthood), which renders 400,000 hits on Google.fr (retrieved 23 April 2009).

16. Interestingly, then, Rousseau is both heir and critic of the attachment parenting tradition, at once counselling women to look to nature for their examples of infant feeding, and denying that a child's 'cues' should be understood as needs for love and comfort.

17. Although, of course, the *Liberté, Egalitié, Fraternité* of the French constitution might be more idealistic than anything else. Indeed, the policy of *not* enforcing positive discrimination on the basis of equality has led to a raw deal for many marginal groups in society.

18. Criticisms of pumping come also from another perspective: it is seen as a way of doubling the labour women have to carry out – to both express and bottle feed – becoming another pressure point for women who can't (or don't want) to breastfeed (Blum 1999).

CONCLUSION

Charlotte: Is there a natural age to wean? Surely we are also cultural beings, which must influence our actions...

Veronika [37, 8-year-old daughter, breastfeeding her 7-year-old daughter, emphasis added]: Well, I guess for me, I don't care what people think of me, which is great, I mean, it makes things a lot easier for me. It means you don't have your life dictated by other people. *Um. I think that regardless of the culture we live in it doesn't change your biological expectations ... every baby on the planet – doesn't matter what they are born into, whether it is royalty or a third world country – every baby is born with the expectation of breastfeeding for anything up to 7 years old. So for me culture ... means nothing. It means nothing, you know.* It just doesn't. And people have to learn to deal with it. I mean if they find it disgusting then they don't have to look.

For the anthropologist, it is always interesting when 'nature' is mobilised in defence of social practices – whether in the realm of parenting practices or elsewhere. Just as interesting, perhaps, is when 'culture' becomes a social object. What happens when mainstream 'culture' is something one's informants reject in the creation of 'natural' countercultures? By way of conclusion, some of these issues are considered.

Through an anthropological engagement with practices of relatedness as critical elements of self-making, it has been argued that 'parenting', as a social activity, needs to be distinguished from the general business of raising children. Mothers (today, in the UK) are expected to do much more than what might once have been considered necessary. This inflation of the parenting role, so reliant on the developmental paradigm, can be read as a symptom of a wider crisis around the social meanings of childhood and adulthood (Lee et al., forthcoming). In an era where children are seen as peculiarly vulnerable and 'at risk', Furedi (2009), for example, recognizes that there has been a concurrent breakdown in adult solidarity. Parents are ever less able to trust other adults in the task of socializing the next generation. This, in turn, has inflated the social role of the mother in particular, both at the level of both policy and of practice, exacerbating a cultural contradiction between the public and private domains.

This volume has explored how a particularly articulate, reflexive sample of mothers have responded to this historical shift by undertaking 'identity work' through mothering practices; that is, it has detailed how one sort of mothering – full-term breastfeeding and attachment parenting – has become central to the construction of these mothers' social selves. They magnify one extreme of the intensive parenting injunction through their long-term, embodied care of their children. At the same time, their position as middle-class consumers (and creators) of ideology means they express what are taken to be general social values about the importance of intensive mothering.

Accountability and the Self

The giving of 'accountability' takes on a particularly moralised edge in the context of mothering, because mothers and children share not one but two bodies (Strathern 2005). To this extent, the child becomes a symbol of maternal devotion and a reflection of her diligence. Mothers do not simply encourage the development of their child's social self through mothering, but develop their own 'selves' in this process.

It is interesting, then, that methods of childcare are so often framed as a play-off between the needs of the mother and those of the child. Once methods of care are defined as either child-centred or mother-centred, then one 'side' logically has to lose out. Accounts of attachment parenting that portray women as sacrificing their 'selves' to be subsumed by the selves of their children are simplistic, and problematic. It seems almost inevitable that by becoming a mother, a woman's 'self' changes. Bristow (2007) comments:

> When individuals become parents they don't subsume themselves but extend themselves – in a sense, they become more than what they were before. The act of raising children, loving them, caring for them, setting them on a trajectory through life, is an act of selfhood, and people do it because they sense it is ultimately more rewarding and meaningful than the accomplishments they might make on their

own, as individuals. To pretend that this impulse isn't there, that as a parent you are doing something despite your own interests rather than because of them, is a dishonest conceit. (Bristow 2007)[1]

Thus 'child-centred' approaches to parenting *can* be understood as part of these mothers' struggle for self-identity, and a prominent part of their identity work as social agents. Attachment mothers experience this process not necessarily as a form of 'oppression' of their individualised selves, but rather as an extension of agency, when understood through the more relational model.

Nevertheless, the attachment mothers here are confronted with a need to justify what is seen to be antisocial behaviour (to use Strathern's definition of society) that in many respects is on the fringes of mainstream patterns of parenting. In narrating their full-term breastfeeding, they employ accountability strategies that work symbiotically to create a vision of motherhood legitimated by a 'natural' basis. It is not simply the case then, that these women are doing what is scientifically 'best'. There is a complex relationship between what 'feels right' to them, and what science says is best for their children. 'Science' or 'evolution' is rarely the ultimate factor in decision-making – though it is notable that in 'choosing health', these women optimise their identities as responsible citizens in a regime of liberal democracy.

In many cases, women in my sample had started breastfeeding their children – or caring for them in an attachment style – because they had read the evidence of its benefits, but over time the science became an ex post facto means of validating choices that 'feel right'. Certainly, as time passes, the fact that breastfeeding 'feels right' is not prioritised in women's accounts, and is typically eclipsed by talk of scientific benefits and evolutionary logic, which are understood as more robust accountability strategies. In the arena of intensive motherhood, it would be a brave mother who declared that she was to breastfeeding to full term simply because it 'felt right'; some cultural scaffolding is typically required. But at the same time, a person's 'feeling' is non-negotiable. Unlike scientific or evolutionary arguments, which are publicly available for deconstruction, women's embodied experiences may be shared (by other breastfeeding mothers), but remain highly personal: the bottom line and, often, last resort in justificatory identity work.

There are interesting ambiguities here then, to the extent that women do not perceive their actions as choices: over time, they understand that they have *no* choice but to parent as they do. To take Strathern's argument again, where maternal selfhood depends on demonstrating the application of one's own knowledge, it would actually be to deny the conditions of one's existence – being a (responsible) mother – not to act in the way that science, or evolution, says is best. Concomitantly, these 'truths' are revealed within women: there is no space for doubt. To question 'gut feelings' would be to deny a fundamental part of oneself.

Making the Choice to Mother

The LLL leaders interviewed in the course of this research insisted that La Leche League was a space for all breastfeeding mothers, but at the same time, many were aware that in the wider community LLL had a reputation for being 'extreme'. In the questionnaire, respondents were asked to comment on how they thought health professionals, other mothers and 'people on the street' saw LLL. The most common answers were (if respondents had even heard of it) that people thought of LLL as some sort of 'cult' that was 'weird', 'extreme', 'hippy' or 'fanatical'. One leader, talking about how LLL was perceived in the wider community, commented:

> *Annette* [*Leader, breastfeeding her 7-year-old son*]: I suppose they probably just think that it is over-zealous really. And, erm, the earth mother sort of thing, of a women who gives all to her children and wastes her own life, because they can't see the value in what the mothers are doing.

Sociologists have noted that one of the enduring features of social groups are their 'commitment mechanisms'. Kanter, who writes about utopian communities in the United States during the 1970s, observes that commitment involves choice (though in this case we may say it is a choice to follow a predetermined pattern). To some extent, the women in my sample are already success stories – unlike others, they have 'persevered' through the often difficult early stages of breastfeeding. At the same time, they need validation of their continuation of breastfeeding. A person's commitment to a choice rests, says Kanter, on knowledge of excluded choices – and a validation of the one that has been made. This is a process that intensifies over time: 'A person becomes increasingly committed both as more of his own internal satisfaction becomes dependent on the group, and his chance to make other choices or pursue other options declines' (Kanter 1972: 70).

Kanter notes that along with other commitment mechanisms, such as sharing food and drink or having ceremonies, the idea of sacrifice and/or renunciation is central to group coherence (Kanter 1972: 72). In the questionnaire, women were asked to list some of the reasons they thought other women did not breastfeed their children. Two thirds of respondents replied that women wanted to breastfeed but were not supported enough, whilst many commented that they probably did not breastfeed because they did not like the dependence of someone else on them. Just over half said it was because they wanted their bodies back for themselves and their partners. Other phrases that arose frequently were that women were 'brainwashed' by formula manufacturers, and 'too selfish' to breastfeed. The following comments were typical:

> *Claire [38, 7-year-old son, breastfeeding 11-month-old son]*: They put themselves before their babies/children but babes only need us like this for a relatively short time overall in breastfeeding, it's no real hardship is it?

> *Debbie [46, 8-year-old son, breastfeeding 4-year-old son]*: A lot of women want a life away from their children and you cannot do both.

Women who have given up careers, as many of my informants had, might be said to have a greater investment in motherhood as a source of identity work than those who have not. Several women pointed out above that work is not possible if one wants to be able to breastfeed to full term (and, we could infer, parent in an attachment parenting style). The implication is that one cannot parent according to a child's needs unless one is also willing to make this sacrifice. These women said, in a joint interview:

> *Lila [37, breastfeeding her 4-year-old son]*: And people make out [breastfeeding] is such a long time, and so tedious, and you think ... it really is not that long a period, it's just a few years.

> *Rachel [41, breastfeeding her 3-year-old son]*: Their IQ and things, it really makes a difference, and I don't think people are aware of those facts ... I think if people knew about it, they would change their attitudes.

> *Lila*: People are more selfish today. People still have this idea of self-sacrifice with breastfeeding.... So they have to promote it in terms of losing weight ... this 'me' thing comes through, they have to watch what they eat, can't drink. People have such a drive towards selfishness.

> *Rachel*: My sister-in-law wanted to go out drinking! So she stopped at six months!

> *Lila*: People have such a drive for individuality. They see it as a sacrifice. People don't see that investing now will save time later. It is a

fraction of their lives. It is just too much for people. People find it too hard to not watch telly, or not have something for a few days. We can't deal with not having things now. Everything is a race.... Other people are too selfish to mother like we do – we are all too much part of the 'me' generation.

Passionate Attachments

Butler (1997) calls attention to processes of subjectivisation, arguing that as a form of power subjection is 'paradoxical' because one is dependent on that subjection for one's very existence. Being a subject, for the women who are reflexive about their identities as mothers, is precisely about *managing* 'our fundamental dependency on a discourse we never chose but that paradoxically, initiates and sustains our agency' (Butler 1997: 2); creating what she calls 'passionate attachments' to our identities. The defensive reactions to those who question the orthodoxy of 'breast is best' are evidence of how passionate the attachment to an 'attachment parenting' identity is. Desiring the subjection is not the fault of the person who does it, but rather an effect of power itself. As Butler puts it, it is not that one 'requires the recognition of the other, and that a form of recognition is conferred through subordination, but rather that one is dependent on power for one's very formation, that that formation is possible without dependency, and that the posture of the adult subject consists precisely in the denial and re-enactment of this dependency' (Butler 1997: 9).

These processes do not occur in a vacuum, of course. Women learn the 'truths' about mothering in a social environment, where certain social values are created and sustained. Sally speaks about 'finding her tribe', who share certain 'norms' about what the mothering relationship should look like. These norms, like any norms, are coercive in that they form the basis of evaluating our conformity (and comfort) in the social nexus. Many norms about mothering can exist in parallel – until one set of norms is held to be better than another. Despite the discourse of choice, the reality is that my informants consider their way of mothering to be optimal, and since it is apparently backed up by science there is little space for disagreement here.

A prominent thread running throughout this book is the difference between description and prescription. In challenging the leap between the two, the analysis points to the aspects of the intensive mothering ideology that are most taken for granted: that the activity of raising children must be child-centred and emotionally absorbing on the part of the mother. A historical and geographical comparison reveals that this is not necessarily the case.

For attachment mothers, information is translated into prescription as a means of validating their own behaviour. Whilst the constitutive effect of norms pulls groups closer in some respects, on a broader scale it can have a divisive effect. It was certainly the case that some attachment mothers made other mothers feel uncomfortable. One particular woman, who is profiled here by way of a postscript, says that although she was 'very pro all the natural stuff' and breastfed each of her children for a year, she found La Leche League meetings an exclusionary space:

> *Sarah [breastfed both daughters for a year]*: I didn't carry on with it, [going to LLL] because I felt a bit uncomfortable with the attitudes towards breastfeeding at that point ... to be honest I felt like it was a bit militant, erm, and righteous. Um. And I mean I don't want to devalue their work because they have been very very valuable to lots of women and I do feel breastfeeding has to be pushed, but I feel that if it comes to the point where the mother is so deeply unhappy that she can't bond with her child at all, well, maybe its not such a sin that a child has the formula. I don't know, I mean, if you try and you really give it a go, and you have good advice, and you give it a good run, I do think it is justified to do something different, but I didn't feel like that was an accepted position there.

She continued, saying that it was the actual interactions in the group that eventually led her to stop coming:

> ...there was this one person there that I found a bit difficult, because, well, for two reasons. Firstly, she was doing extended breastfeeding, which, I'm kind of OK with ... but because the older child was being quite rude in stealing my daughter's sandwiches, which I wouldn't have minded if the mother had done something about it, or if it had just been once or something, but nothing happened. And I just felt like this child just wasn't very disciplined. Not that I think children should be under an iron grip, but to a certain extent I think it is the parent's responsibility to make sure the child behaves in a reasonable way, so you know, take the sandwich and say 'don't take this, perhaps you can share it' or something. So I don't know, I just sort of found it a bit off-putting.... But mainly I just didn't carry on because I guess I didn't see myself as that radical about it. So yeah I do think it is really important, and I would encourage anyone to do it, because once you get it, it can be quite enjoyable, it's quite a wonderful experience, I am really glad I did it, but I don't feel astronomic about it.

The 'militancy' that Sarah perceived in the group did not echo her own feelings about breastfeeding, so she was happy not to return, despite continuing to breastfeed her children: for her, full-term breastfeeding was not the central element of her identity work as a mother. One mother's trailblazing is another's 'spoiling for a fight':

> ... at the time it was a bit of a 'hoo-haa' because someone wanted to breastfeed in the House of Commons ... and so that was the discussion at this meeting, and I just sort of felt like it was ... you know, spoiling for a fight. 'We are going to breastfeed our children right outside all day' and like 'strike'! and it was a bit humorous ... but they weren't being humorous, and so I don't know, in a way I'm being a bit negative, because I think public attitudes to breastfeeding issues need to be confronted, but I just didn't feel like I was the person to do it, so I just felt a bit uncomfortable.

It seems ironic, then, that intensive parenting – of which attachment mothering is but one expression – aims to bring about stronger social ties, because in fact the ethos can pit groups of women against each other (those who do it 'right', those who do it 'wrong'). Infant feeding operates as a particularly moralised barometer of this antagonism: the women who do not breastfeed in the early days mirror the mothers who do breastfeed in the later ones, as both of them face public scrutiny and opprobrium. This climate has created a situation where mothers feel less certain of their ability to turn to each other for support in the general business of raising children (Lee and Bristow 2009). Instead, the 'tribe' that does it 'right' is pushed further inward, away from society, identifying others 'out there' not as partners in a shared endeavour of community building, but as victims in need of education. As one woman says:

> *Questionnaire*: Please say how explaining your decisions to other people about how you feed your infant makes you feel, as a mother:
>
> *Debbie* [*46, 8-year-old son, breastfeeding 4-year-old son*]: I have lost a lot of friends and feel I am in a bubble world. I can only relate to others who have mothered the same.

Notes

1. Of course, Bristow's comment can only be understood in the context of widely available contraception and abortion.

Appendix 1

**Short Term and Long Term Health Benefits
of Breast Feeding for the Child and Mother
in Developed Countries**[1]

CI=confidence interval; OR=odds ratio.

Short term and long term health benefits of breast feeding for the child in developed countries

Condition	Incidence or risk reduction	Studies included	Comment
Gastrointestinal infection	Reduced risk of diarrhoea in 1st year for infants who were breast fed compared with those who were not (OR 0.36, 95% CI 0.18 to 0.74)[i]	1 systematic review of 14 cohort studies and 3 case control studies	Risk reduction taken from 1 case-control study only; few studies controlled for potential confounders
Lower respiratory tract diseases	Reduced risk of hospital admission for respiratory disease in term infants <1 year who were exclusively breast fed for >4 months compared with those who were formula fed (OR 0.28, 95% CI 0.14 to 0.54)[i]	Meta-analysis of 7 cohort studies	Good quality meta-analysis with adjustment for potential confounders
Acute otitis media	Reduced risk when comparing ever breast fed with never breast fed (OR 0.77, 95% CI 0.64 to 0.91) and exclusive breast feeding for >3 months with never breast fed (0.50, 0.36 to 0.70)[i]	5 cohort studies and 1 case-control study	Studies were of moderate or poor quality; potential confounders were not considered in some studies
High blood pressure	Reduction of <1.5 mm Hg in systolic and <0.5 mm Hg in diastolic blood pressure in adults who were ever breast fed compared with formula fed[i]; reduction of 1.21 mm Hg (95% CI to 1.72 to −0.70) in systolic and 0.49 mm Hg (−0.87 to −0.11) in diastolic blood pressure in adults who were ever breast fed compared with formula fed[ii]	Two meta-analyses evaluated 26 studies, with 13 studies common to both[1]; meta-analysis of 30 mostly cohort and cross sectional studies[2]	Duration and exclusivity of breast feeding varied; age ranged from 1 to 71 years; publication bias and residual confounding are possible

Condition	Incidence or risk reduction	Studies included	Comment
Total cholesterol	0.18 mmol/l and 0.2 mmol/l reduction in total and low density lipoprotein cholesterol in adults who were ever breast fed compared with formula fed: 0.18 mmol/l (95% CI −0.30 to −0.06) reduction in mean total cholesterol in adults who were ever breast fed compared with formula fed[ii]	1 meta-analysis of 37 cohort and case-control studies[i]; 1 meta-analysis with 28 estimates of total cholesterol from 23 cohort studies and cross sectional studies[ii]	Analyses of potential confounders, particularly age and fasting status, varied: no significant effect was seen in children or adolescents
Overweight and obesity	Reduced risk of obesity in adolescence or as an adult for ever breast fed compared with never breast fed (OR 0.76, 95% CI 0.67 to 0.86 and 0.93, 0.88 to 0.99) in two meta-analyses; a third meta-regression found a 4% risk reduction (unadjusted OR 0.96/month of breast feeding, 0.94 to 0.98) of being overweight in adult life for each additional month of any breast feeding in infancy[i]; people who had ever been breast fed were less likely to be overweight or obese as adults (0.78, 0.72 to 0.84)[ii]	Two meta-analyses of 9 and 17 cohort studies or cross sectional studies and one systematic review using meta-regression of 28 cohort or cross sectional studies[i]; meta-analysis of 33 mainly cohort studies or cross sectional studies[ii]	Weight was examined at different time points; not all potential confounders were adjusted for; larger studies controlling for socioeconomic status and parental anthropometry showed a statistically significant protective effect, making confounding and publication bias less likely

Condition	Incidence or risk reduction	Studies included	Comment
Type 1 diabetes	Any breast feeding for >3 months compared with breast feeding <3 months reduced the risk of childhood type 1 diabetes (OR 0.81, 95% CI 0.74 to 0.89 and 0.88, 0.81 to 0.96)[i]	Two meta-analyses of 18 and 17 case-control studies	Not all confounders were adjusted for and exclusivity of breast feeding varied; 5 of 6 subsequent studies report similar results
Type 2 diabetes	Any breast feeding reduced the risk in later life compared with exclusive formula feeding (OR 0.61, 95% CI 0.44 to 0.85[i] and 0.63, 0.45 to 0.89)[2]	Meta-analysis of 7 mostly cohort and cross sectional studies[i]; meta-analysis of 5 cohort studies[ii]	Not all primary studies adjusted for all important confounders and publication bias is possible
Necrotising enterocolitis	Reduced risk when comparing breast milk with formula milk in preterm births (risk ratio 0.42, 95% CI 0.18 to 0.96)[i]	Meta-analysis of 4 trials in pre-term infants (n=1134)	Gestational age ranged from 23 to 33 weeks and birth weight from <1 kg to >1.6 kg
Childhood leukaemias	Any breast feeding for at least 6 months reduced the risk of acute lymphocytic leukaemia (OR 0.80, 95% CI 0.71 to 0.91) and acute myelogenous leukaemia (0.85, 0.73 to 0.98)[i]	One meta-analysis of 14 case-control studies	The included studies were of good or moderate quality
Pain during procedures	Breast feeding or supplemental breast milk alleviated pain during a single painful procedure compared with placebo or positioning or no intervention[v]	Systematic review of 11 randomised or quasi-randomised controlled trials of term infants (n=10 300)	Studies varied in the control used and in both physiological and behavioural pain assessment measures

Condition	Incidence or risk reduction	Studies included	Comment
Atopic dermatitis	Reduced risk comparing children with a family history of atopy exclusively breast fed >3 months with those breast fed for <3 months (OR 0.58, 95% CI 0.41 to 0.92)[i]	1 meta-analysis of 18 prospective cohort studies	Heterogeneity in age of onset and duration of atopic dermatitis
Childhood asthma	Reduced risk for infants without a family history of asthma in children <10 who were breast fed (mixed or exclusive) for >3 months compared with those who were not breast fed (OR 0.74, 95% CI 0.60 to 0.94)[i]; conflicting evidence for infants with a family history of asthma	Meta-analysis of 12 prospective cohort studies with a mean follow-up of 4.1 years; 10 prospective cohort studies	Equivocal conclusions from more recently published studies of moderate quality; relation between breast feeding and risk of asthma in older children is unclear
Cognitive development in infants	No definitive conclusion in term or preterm infants[i]; performance in childhood intelligence tests was higher in those breast fed for >1 month (mean difference 4.9, 95% CI 2.97 to 6.92)[iii]	3 meta-analyses of 40, 24, and 11 mostly cohort studies, 7 subsequent cohort studies, and 1 secondary analysis in term infants; 8 cohort studies in preterm infants[i]; meta-analysis of 7 higher quality cohort studies and one randomised controlled trial[iii]	Not all primary studies adjusted for maternal education or intelligence, which reduces the advantage from breast feeding
Sudden infant death syndrome	Any breast feeding was associated with a reduction in risk compared with exclusive formula feeding (OR 0.64, 95% CI 0.51 to 0.81)[i]	One meta-analysis of 7 case-control studies fitting strict selection criteria	Essential requirements: autopsy confirmed diagnosis, adjustment for sleeping positions, maternal smoking, socioeconomic status

Short term and long term health benefits of breast feeding for mothers in developed countries (iii, iv)

Condition	Incidence or risk reduction	Studies included	Comment
Breast cancer	Reduced risk of 4.3% for each year of breast feeding in one meta-analysis and 28% reduction for >12 months' breast feeding in another[i]; 1 of the meta-analyses and the systematic review reported decreased risk mainly in premenopausal women	Two meta-analyses and 1 systematic review of 47, 23, and 27 cohort and case control studies	No studies evaluated exclusive breast feeding; 3 primary studies published subsequently report consistent findings
Ovarian cancer	Any breast feeding was associated with a reduced risk of ovarian cancer compared with never breast feeding (OR 0.79, 95% CI 0.68 to 0.91)[i]	Meta-analysis of 9 case-control studies	Moderate and poor quality studies with inconsistent reporting of breast feeding
Type 2 diabetes	For women without a history of gestational diabetes, each additional year of breast feeding was associated with a reduced risk (OR 0.63, 95% CI 0.54 to 0.73 in one cohort; 0.76, 0.71 to 0.81 in the other)[i]	Two large cohorts from the USA nurses health study, one prospective (n=83 585) and one retrospective (n=73 418)	In women with a history of gestational diabetes, breast feeding had no significant effect
Postnatal depression	Three studies found an association between early cessation of breast feeding or not breast feeding and an increased risk of postnatal depression[i]; cause and effect cannot be determined	Six prospective cohort studies (n=5524)	Studies of moderate or poor quality; no studies screened for depression at baseline; unclear definitions of breast feeding

Notes

1. Reproduced from Hoddinott, Tappin and Wright (2008), drawing on (i):
   Ip et al. (2007); (ii); Horta et al. (2007); (iii) Edmond and Bahl (2006);
   (iv) Henderson, Anthony and McGuire (2007); (v) Shah, Aliwalas and
   Shah (2006), all included in References.

APPENDIX 2

Summary of Demographic Results from Questionnaire Responses

Sample (size)	UK (25)	France (19)	Anglophone (4)
Average age (median)	• 35	• 33	• 35
Marital status	• 76% Married • 16% Cohab • 8% Single	• 74% Married • 21% Cohab • 5% Single	• 75% Married • 25% Single
Education	• 20% P/Grad • 64% Degree • 8% A levels • 8% GCSE	• 84% P/Grad • 16% Degree[1]	• 25% P/Grad • 50% Degree • 25% A levels
Employment	• 4% F/Time • 32% P/Time • 16% M/Leave • 48% Not Work	• 37% F/Time • 26% P/Time • 16% M/Leave • 21% Not Work	• 75% P/T • 25% M/Leave
Ethnicity (self-defined)	• 88% British • 12% Other	• Unclear %[2]	• 75% White • 25% Indian
Parity	• 52% 1 child • 36% 2 children • 12% 3 children	• 68% 1 child • 26% 2 children • 5% 3 children	• 75% 1 child • 25% 2 children
Age range of children breastfed	• 0 months– 4 years, 6 months	• 0 months– 3 years, 8 months	• 4 months– 5 years, 2 months
Average age of children breastfed	• 18 months	• 9 months	• 9 months
Child sex	• 50% Female • 50% Male	• 50% Female • 50% Male	• 75% Female • 25% Male

Notes

1. The meaning of 'degree' is not culturally stable and was classified by some of my French informants to mean graduation from high school, thus many more listed postgraduate qualifications than in the UK.
2. Many women in France wrote that this was not a question they were happy to answer. The vast majority of those who did answer wrote that they were white Europeans.

References

Aegnst, J. and Layne, L. 2010. '"The Need to Bleed?" A Feminist Technology Assessment of Menstrual-Suppressing Birth Control Pills,' in Layne, L. Vostral, S. and Boyer, K. (eds), *Feminist Technology*. Chicago: University of Illinois Press, pp 55–88.

Ainsworth, M., Andry, R., Harlow, R., Lebovici, S., Mead, M., Prugh, D. and Wotton, B. (eds), 1962. *Deprivation of Maternal Care: A Reassessment of Its Effects*. Geneva: WHO.

Ainsworth, M., Blehar, M., Waters, W. and Wall, S. 1978. *Patterns of Attachment: A Psychological Study of the Strange Situation*. Hillsdale, NJ: Lawrence Erlbaum.

Allsop, J. Jones, K. and Baggott, R. 2004. 'Health Consumer Groups in the UK: A New Social Movement?' *Sociology of Health & Illness* 26(6): 737–756.

American Academy of Pediatrics. 1984. 'Report of the Task Force on the Assessment of the Scientific Evidence Relating to Infant-Feeding Practices and Infant Health', *Pediatrics* 74(4) (supp.): 579–584.

American Academy of Pediatrics. 1997. 'Breastfeeding and the Use of Human Milk', *Pediatrics* 100 (6): 1035–1039.

American Institute for Cancer Research. 2008. *Food, Nutrition, Physical Activity and the Prevention of Cancer: A Global Perspective*. Retrieved 24 April 2008 from http://www.aicr.org/site/PageServer?pagename=res_report_second

Andrews, F. 1991. 'Controlling Motherhood: Observations on the Culture of La Leche League', *Canadian Review of Sociology and Anthropology* 28(1): 84–98.

API (Attachment Parenting International). 2009. 8 Principles of AP. Retrieved 23 March 2009 http://www.attachmentparenting.org/principles/principles.php

Apple, R. 1987. *Mothers and Medicine: A Social History of Infant Feeding 1890–1950*. Madison, WI: University of Wisconsin Press.

Apple, R. 1995. 'Constructing Mothers: Scientific Motherhood in the Nineteenth and Twentieth Centuries', *Social History of Medicine* 8(2): 161–178.

Apple, R. 2006. *Perfect Motherhood: Science and Childrearing in America*. New Brunswick, NJ, and London: Rutgers University Press.

Arendell, T. 2000. 'Conceiving and Investigating Motherhood: The Decade's Scholarship', *Journal of Marriage and the Family* 62(November): 1192–1207.

Ariès, P. 1962. *Centuries of Childhood; A Social History of Family Life*. New York: Vintage Books.

Avishai, O. 2007. 'Managing the Lactating Body: The Breast-Feeding Project and Privileged Motherhood', *Qualitative Sociology* 30: 135–152.

Avishai, O. 2010. 'Managing the Lactating Body: The Breastfeeding Project in the Age of Anxiety', in Liamputtong, P. (ed.), *Infant Feeding Practices: A Cross-Cultural Perspective*. London: Springer, pp. 23–39.

Badinter, E. 1981 [1980]. *The Myth of Motherhood: A Historical View of the Maternal Instinct*, trans. Roger De Garis. London: Souvenir Press.

Badinter, E. 2010. *Le conflit : La femme et la mere*. Paris: Flammarion.

Ball, H. 2007. 'Bed-Sharing Practices of Initially Breastfed Infants in the First 6 Months of Life', *Infant and Child Development* 16(4): 387–401.

Baraitser, L. 2006. 'Oi Mother, Keep Ye' Hair On! Impossible Transformations of Maternal Subjectivity', *Studies in Gender and Sexuality* 7(3): 217–238.

Battersby, S. 2006. 'Exploring Attitudes towards Infant Feeding', in Dykes, F. and Hall-Moran, V. (eds), *Maternal and Infant Nutrition and Nurture Controversies and Challenges*. London: Quay Books, pp. 204–232.

BBC. 2007. 'Gang Crime 'Due To Absent Dads'.' Retrieved 1 April 2011 from http://news.bbc.co.uk/1/hi/uk_politics/6956303.stm

Beck, U. and Beck-Gernsheim, E. 1995. *The Normal Chaos of Love*. Oxford: Polity Press.

Bell, S. 2004. 'Intensive Performances of Mothering: A Sociological Perspective', *Qualitative Research* 4(1): 45–75.

Bengson, D. 1999. *How Weaning Happens*. Schaumburg, IL: LLLI.

Bernshaw, N. 1991. 'Does Breastfeeding Protect Against Sudden Infant Death Syndrome?' *Journal of Human Lactation* 7(2): 73–79.

Birch, E., Birch, D., Hoffman, D., Hale, L., Everett, M. and Uauy, R. 1993. 'Breast-feeding and Optimal Visual Development', *Journal of Pediatric Ophthalmol Strabismus* 30: 33–38.

Birth Choice UK. 2011. Home Birth Rates Retrieved 14 December 2011 from http://www.birthchoiceuk.com/BirthChoiceUKFrame.htm?http://www.birthchoiceuk.com/HomeBirthRates.htm

Bitoun, P. 1994. 'The Economic Value of Breastfeeding', *Les Dossiers de l'Obstétrique* 216: 12–13.

Blackburn, S. 2000. *Being Good: A Short Introduction to Ethics*. Oxford: Oxford University Press.

Blaffer Hrdy, S. 2000. *Mother Nature: Maternal Instincts and the Shaping of the Species*. London: Vintage.

Bloch, M. 1989. *Ritual, History and Power: Selected Papers in Anthropology*. London: Athlone.

Blum, L. 1999. *At the Breast: Ideologies of Breastfeeding and Motherhood in the Contemporary United States*. Boston: Beacon Press.

Blum, L. and Vandewater, E. 1993. 'Mothers Construct Fathers: Destabilized Patriarchy in La Leche League', *Qualitative Sociology* 16(1): 3–22.

Bobel, C. 2001. 'Bounded Liberation: A Focused Study of La Leche League', *Gender & Society* 15: 131–152.

Bobel, C. 2002. *The Paradox of Natural Mothering.* Philadelphia: Temple University Press.

Bowlby, J. 1969. *Attachment.* London: Pelican.

Bowlby, J. 1995 [1952]. *Maternal Care and Mental Health.* Lanham, MD: Jason Aronson.

Bowlby, J. 2005 [1988]. *A Secure Base: Clinical Applications of Attachment Theory.* London: Routledge.

Breastfeeding Manifesto Coalition. 2007. Breastfeeding Manifesto. Retrieved 3 December 2008 from http://www.breastfeedingmanifesto.org.uk/

Bristow, J. 2007. 'Lesson 1: It's Not All About You', in *Jennie Bristow's Guide for Subversive Parents.* Retrieved 15 May 2007 from http://www.spiked-online.com/index.php?/site/issues/C109/

Broadfoot, M., Britten, J., Tappin, D. and MacKenzie, J. 2005. 'The Baby Friendly Hospital Initiative and Breastfeeding Rates in Scotland', *Archives of Disease in Childhood, Fetal and Neonatal Edition* 90: F114–F116.

Brown, M. 1982. 'Corticotropin-Releasing Factor: Actions on the Sympathetic Nervous System and Metabolism', *Endocrinology* 111: 928–931.

Brubaker, R. and Cooper, F. 2000. 'Beyond "Identity"', *Theory and Society* 29: 1–47.

Buckley, K. 2001. 'Long-Term Breastfeeding: Nourishment or Nurturance?' *Journal of Human Lactation* 17(4): 304–312.

Buskens, P. 2001. 'The Impossibility of "Natural Parenting" for Modern Mothers: On Social Structure and the Formation of Habit', *Association for Research on Mothering Journal* 3(1): 75–86.

Butler, J. 1997. *The Psychic Life of Power: Studies in Subjection.* Stanford, CA: Stanford University Press.

Butler, N. and Golding, J. 1986. *From Birth to Five: A Study of the Health and Behaviour of Britain's Five Year Olds.* Oxford: Pergamon Press.

Cahill, M. 2001. *Seven Voices, One Dream.* Schaumburg, IL: La Leche League International.

Carsten, J. (ed.). 2000. *Cultures of Relatedness: New Approaches to the Study of Kinship.* Cambridge: Cambridge University Press.

Carter, P. 1995. *Feminism, Breasts and Breast-Feeding.* Hampshire and London: Macmillan Press.

Chandra, R. 1997. 'Five Year Follow-up of High Risk Infants with Family History of Allergy Who Were Exclusively Breastfed or Fed Partial Whey Hydrolysate, Soy and Conventional Cows' Milk Formulas', *Journal of Paediatric Gastro-Enterology and Nutrition* 24: 380–388.

Clarke, A. 2007. 'Consuming Children and Making Mothers: Birthday Parties, Gifts and the Pursuits of Sameness', *Hoizontes Antropoliogicos* 13(28): 263–287.

Clayton, F., Sealy, J. and Pfeiffer, S. 2006. 'Weaning Age among Foragers at Matjes River Rock Shelter, South Africa, from Stable Nitrogen and Carbon Isotope Analysis', *American Journal of Physical Anthropology* 129(2): 311–317.

Clifford, J. and Marcus, G. 1986. Writing Culture: The Poetics and Politics of Ethnography. Berkeley: University of California Press.

Clough, P. and Halley, J. (eds). 2007. *The Affective Turn: Theorizing the Social.* London: Duke University Press.

Comaroff, J. and Comaroff, J. 1991. *Of Revelation and Revolution.* Chicago: University of Chicago Press.

Commings, R. and Klineberg R. 1993. 'Breastfeeding and Other Reproductive Factors in the Risk of Hip Fracture in Elderly Women', *International Journal of Epidemiology* 2(4): 684–691.

Commons Leader. 2009. *Right to Breastfeed Act.* Retrieved 23 March 2009 from www.commonsleader.gov.uk/OutPut/page2438.asp now http://www.adviceguide.org.uk/england/discrimination_e/discrimination_about_discrimination_e/equality_act_2010_discrimination_and_your_rights.htm

Connolly, W. 1999. *Why I Am Not a Secularist.* London: University of Minnesota Press.

Corsín Jiménez, A. 2007. 'Industry Going Public: Rethinking Knowledge and Administration', in Edwards, J., Harvey, P. and Wade, P. (eds), *Anthropology and Science: Epistemologies in Practice.* Oxford and New York: Berg, pp. 39–57.

Crossley, M.L. 2009. 'Breastfeeding as a Moral Imperative: An Autoethnographic Study', *Feminism and Psychology* 19: 71–87.

Cunningham, A., Jelliffe, D. and Jelliffe, E. 1991. 'Breast-Feeding and Health in the 1980s: A Global Epidemiologic Review', *Journal of Pediatrics* 118(5): 659–666.

Damasio, A. 2006 [1994]. *Descartes' Error: Emotion, Reason and the Human Brain.* London: Vintage Books.

Davis, D. and Bell, P. 1991. 'Infant Feeding Practices and Occlusal Outcomes: A Longitudinal Study', *Journal of the Canadian Dental Association* 57(7): 593–594.

Davis-Floyd, R. and Davis, E. 1997. 'Intuition as Authoritative Knowledge in Midwifery and Home Birth', in Davis-Floyd, R. and Sargent, C. (eds), *Childbirth and Authoritative Knowledge: Cross-Cultural Perspectives.* London: University of California Press, pp. 316–349.

Daycare Trust. 2005. *Childcare Costs Surveys.* Retrieved 6 September 2012 from http://www.daycaretrust.org.uk/pages/childcare-costs-surveys.html

Dermott, E. 2008. *Intimate Fatherhood: A Sociological Analysis.* London: Routledge.

Dettwyler, K. 1995. 'A Time to Wean: A Hominid Blueprint for the Natural Age of Weaning', in Stuart-Macadam, P. and Dettwyler, K. (eds), *Breastfeeding: Bio-cultural Perspectives.* New York: Aldine de Gruyter, pp. 167–217.

Dewey, K. 2001. 'Nutrition, Growth, and Complementary Feeding of the Breastfed Infant', *Pediatric Clinics of North America* 48(1): 87–104.

Dewey, K., Heinig, M. and Nommsen, L. 1993. 'Maternal Weight-Loss Patterns During Prolonged Lactation', *American Journal of Clinical Nutrition* 58: 162–168.

DfE (Department for Education). 2011. 'Parenting Classes Trial'. Retrieved 14 December 2011 from http://www.education.gov.uk/childrena ndyoungpeople/families/a00200255/parenting-classes-trial

DfES (Department for Education and Skills). 2003. *Every Child Matters.* Nottingham: DfES Publications.

DfES. 2007. *Every Parent Matters.* Nottingham: DfES Publications.

DH (Department of Health). 2004a. *National Service Framework for Children, Young People and Maternity Services.* London: Department of Health.

DH. 2004b. *Choosing Health.* London: Department of Health. Retrieved 23 March 2009 from www.dh.gov.uk/Publicationsandstatistics/Publications/ PublicationsPolicyAndGuidance/DH_4094550 now http://webarchive .nationalarchives.gov.uk/+/dh.gov.uk/en/publicationsandstatistics/pub lications/publicationspolicyandguidance/dh_4094550

DH. 2005a. *Maternal and Infant Nutrition.* London: Department of Health. Retrieved 7 December 2005 from http://www.dh.gov.uk/PolicyAndGuid ance/HealthAndSocialCareTopics/MaternalAndInfantNutrition/fs/en

DH. 2005b. *Choosing a Better Diet.* London: Department of Health.

DH. 2005c. *National Breastfeeding Awareness Week.* Retrieved 7 December 2005 from http://www.breastfeeding.nhs.uk/nb_nbaw.asp

DH. 2005d. *Infant Feeding Survey 2005.* London: Department of Health. Retrieved 17 September 2008 from http://www.ic.nhs.uk/webfiles/publi cations/breastfeed2005/InfantFeedingSurvey190506_PDF.pdf

DH. 2011. *Statistical release: Breastfeeding initiation and prevalence at 6 to 8 weeks - Quarter 3, 2010/11.* Retrieved 21 March 2011 from http://www.dh.gov .uk/en/Publicationsandstatistics/Statistics/StatisticalWorkAreas/Statisti calpublichealth/DH_124340

Directgov. 2011. Pregnancy and Maternity rights. Retrieved 13 April 2011 from http://webarchive.nationalarchives.gov.uk/+/www.direct.gov.uk/en/ Parents/Moneyandworkentitlements/WorkAndFamilies/Pregnancyan dmaternityrights/DG_10029285 now https://www.gov.uk/maternity-leave

Douglas, M. 1986. *How Institutions Think.* Syracuse, NY: Syracuse University Press.

Douglas, S. and Michaels, M. 2004. *The Mommy Myth: The Idealization of Motherhood and How It Has Undermined All Women.* New York: Free Press.

Dowling, S. 2009a. 'Women's Experiences of Long-Term Breastfeeding', *The Practising Midwife* 12(10): 22–25.

Dowling S. 2009b. 'Inside Information: Researching Long-Term Breastfeeding', *The Practising Midwife* 12(11): 22–26.

Ducey, A. 2007. 'More Than a Job: Meaning, Affect and Training Health Care Workers', in Clough, P. and Halley, J. (eds), *The Affective Turn: Theorizing the Social.* London: Duke University Press, pp. 187–208.

Duncan, B., Ey, J., Holberg, C., Wright, A., Martinez, F. and Taussig, L. 1993. 'Exclusive Breastfeeding for at Least 4 months Protects against Otitis Media', *Paediatrics* 91(5): 867–872.

Duncan, S., Edwards, R., Reynolds, T. and Allred, P. 2003. 'Mothering, Paid Work and Partnering: Values and Theories', *Work Employment & Society* 17(2): 309–330.

Dupuis, M. 2002. *Nature's Perfect Food: How Milk Became America's Drink.* New York: New York University Press.

Dyson, L., Renfrew, M., McFadden, A., McCormick, F., Herbert, G. and Thomas, J. 2006. *Promotion of Breastfeeding Initiation and Duration: Evidence into Practice Briefing.* London: National Institute for Clinical Excellence.

Earle, S. 2002. 'Factors Affecting the Initiation of Breastfeeding: Implications for Breastfeeding Promotion', *Health Promotion International* 17(3): 205–214.

Edmond, K. and Bahl, R. 2006. *Optimal Feeding of Low-Birth-Weight Infants: Technical Review.* Geneva: WHO. Retrieved 1 April 2009 from http://whqlibdoc.who.int/publications/2006/9789241595094_eng.pdf

Edwards, R. (2002) 'Conceptualising relationships between home and school in children's lives' in Edwards, R. (ed). *Children, Home and School: Regulation, Autonomy or Connection?* London: Routledge Falmer.

Elle. 2008. 'Quand Superwoman Rentre à la Maison'. Retrieved 23 April 2009 from http://www.elle.fr/elle/societe/les-enquetes/quand-super-woman-rentre-a-la-maison/la-fin-du-feminisme/(gid)/740943

Engels, F. 1972 [1884]. *The Origin of the Family, Private Property and the State.* New York: Pathfinder.

Erikson, E. 1959. *Identity and the Life Cycle.* New York: International Universities Press.

Esping-Anderson, G. (1999) *Social Foundations of Post-industrial Economics,* Oxford: OUP.

Eyer, D. 1992. *Mother-Infant Bonding: A Scientific Fiction.* New Haven, CT, and London: Yale University Press.

Faircloth, C. Hoffman, D and Layne, L. (Eds). Forthcoming. *Parenting in Global Perspective: Negotiating Ideologies of Kinship, Self and Politics.* Routledge.

Featherstone. B. 2009. *Contemporary Fathering: Theory, Policy and Practice.* Bristol: The Policy Press.

Fildes, V. 1986. *Breasts, Bottles, and Babies: A History of Infant Feeding.* Edinburgh: Edinburgh University Press.

Fitzpatrick, M. 2004. *MMR and Autism: What Parents Need to Know.* London: Routledge.

Food Standards Agency. 2009. *Consultation on the Panel's Draft Report on Infant Formula and Follow-On Formula and Material Considered by the Review Panel.* Retrieved 13 April 2011 from http://collections.europarchive.org/tna/20100927130941/http://food.gov.uk/healthiereating/nutcomms/infformreview/paneldraftreport

Franklin, S. 1990. 'Review: *Primate Visions: Gender, Race and Nature in the World of Modern Science* by Donna Haraway', *Journal of the History of Sexuality* 1(2): 338–340.

Franklin, S. and McKinnon, S. (eds). 2001. *Relative Values: Reconfiguring Kinship Studies*. London: Duke University Press.

Freud, S. 1977 [1910]. 'A Special Type of Choice of Object Made by Men (Contributions to the Psychology of Love 1)', in Richards, A. and Dickinson, A. (eds.), *On Sexuality: The Penguin Freud Library*. London: Penguin Books, vol. 7, pp. 227–242.

Furedi, F. 2002. *Paranoid Parenting: Why Ignoring the Experts May Be Best for Your Child*. Chicago: Chicago Review Press.

Furedi, F. 2005. 'Taking the Social Out of Policy: A Critique of the Politics of Behaviour', *Diverse Britain: Social Practice and Social Policy*. Retrieved 1 May 2007 from http://www.lsbu.ac.uk/families/conference06/TakingthesocialoutofpolicyFF.pdf (Expired)

Furedi, F. 2008. 'Frank Furedi's Really Bad Ideas: Politicising Science', *Spiked-online* (15 January). Retrieved 6 April 2008 from http://www.spiked-online.com/index.php?/site/article/4275/

Furedi, F. 2009. *Wasted: Why education isn't educating*. London: Continuum.

Gardner, R. 1997. 'The Embedment-in-the-Brain-Circuitry Phenomenon: Implications', *Journal of the American Academy of Psychoanalysis* 25: 151–176.

Gerhardt, S. 2004. *Why Love Matters: How Affection Shapes a Baby's Brain*. London: Routledge.

Giddens, A. 1991. *Modernity and Self-Identity: Self and Society in the Late Modern Age*. Cambridge: Polity.

Gillman, M., Rifas-Shiman, S., Camargo, C., Berkey, C., Frazier, A., Rockett, H., Field, A. and Colditz, G. 2001. 'Risk of Being Overweight Among Adolescents Who Were Breastfed as Infants', *Journal of the American Medical Association* 285: 2461–2467.

Ginsburg, F. and Rapp, R. (eds). 1995. *Conceiving the New World Order: The Global Politics of Reproduction*. London: University of California Press.

Goffman, E. 1959. *The Presentation of Self in Everyday Life*. New York: Doubleday.

Goldman, A. 1993. 'The Immune System of Human Milk: Antimicrobial, Anti-inflammatory and Immunomodulating Properties', *The Pediatric Infectious Disease Journal* 12(8): 664–671.

Goldman, A., Garsa, C. and Goldblum, R. 1983. 'Immunologic Components in Human Milk During Weaning', *Acta Paediatrica Scandinavica* 72(1): 133–134.

Goody, E. 1982. *Parenthood and Social Reproduction: Fostering and Occupational Roles in West Africa*. Cambridge: Cambridge University Press.

Gorham, H. and Andrews, F. 1990. 'La Leche League: A Feminist Perspective', in Arnup, K., Levesque, A. and Pierson, R. (eds), *Delivering Motherhood*. New York: Routledge, pp. 238–269.

Guardian. 2010. French Philosopher Says Feminism Under Threat from 'Good Motherhood'. Retrieved 11 March 2010 from http://www.guard ian.co.uk/world/2010/feb/12/france-feminism-elisabeth-badinter

Guardian Forum. 2010. *Making Babies in the 21st Century: The Rise of Reproductive Technologies.* 2 November 2010. Retrieved 13 March 2011 from http://www.gender.cam.ac.uk/events/guardianforum/

Gulick, E. 1986. 'The Effects of Breastfeeding on Toddler Health', *Pediatric Nursing* 12(1): 51–54.

Hampshire, S. 2005. *Living and Working in France.* London: Survival Books.

Haraway, D. 1978a. 'Animal Sociology and a Natural Economy of the Body Politic. Part I: A Political Physiology of Dominance', *Signs* 4(1) ('Women, Science and Society'): 21–36.

Haraway, D. 1978b. 'Animal Sociology and a Natural Economy of the Body Politic. Part II: The Past Is the Contested Zone: Human Nature and Theories of Production and Reproduction in Primate Behavior Studies', *Signs* 4(1) ('Women, Science and Society'): 37–60.

Haraway, D. 1988. 'Situated Knowledges: The Science Question in Feminism and the Privilege of Partial Perspective', *Feminist Studies* 14(3): 575–599.

Haraway, D. 1989. *Primate Visions: Gender, Race and Nature in the World of Modern Science.* New York: Routledge.

Hardyment, C. 1995. *Perfect Parents: Baby-Care Advice Past and Present.* Oxford: Oxford University Press.

Hardyment, C. 2007. *Dream Babies: Childcare Advice from John Locke to Gina Ford.* London: Francis Lincoln.

Hausman, B. 2003. *Mother's Milk: Breastfeeding Controversies in American Culture.* London: Routledge.

Hays, S. 1996. *The Cultural Contradictions of Motherhood.* New Haven, CT, and London: Yale University Press.

Head, E. 2011. 'Don't Rush to Mush? Infants, Food and Contemporary Feeding Practices', *Feeding Children in the New Parenting Culture* 21 March 2010, British Library, Organized by the Centre for Parenting Culture Studies. Retrieved 4 August 2010 from http://blogs.kent.ac.uk/parentingculturestudies/pcs-events/previous-events/feeding-children/abstracts-and-papers/

Henderson, G., Anthony, M. and McGuire, W. 2007. 'Formula Milk versus Maternal Breast Milk for Feeding Preterm or Low Birth Weight Infants', *Cochrane Database Systematic Review* 4: CD002972.

Hess, E. 1966. 'Imprinting', in King, R. (ed.), *Readings for an Introduction to Psychology.* McGraw-Hill: New York, pp. 39–46.

Hoddinott, P., Tappin, D. and Wright, C. 2008. 'Clinical Review: Breastfeeding', *British Medical Journal* 336(April): 881–887.

Hoffman, D. 2003. 'Childhood Ideology in the United States: A Comparative Cultural View', *International Review of Education* 49(1–2): 191–211.

Hoffman, D. 2008. 'The Possible Future of a Critical Anthropology of Parenting', *Annual Meeting of the American Anthropological Association,* San Francisco, CA, November, 19–23, 2008.

Horta, B., Bahl, R., Martines, J. and Victora, C. 2007. *Evidence of the Long-Term Effects of Breastfeeding.* Geneva: WHO. Retrieved 1 October 2008 from http://whqlibdoc.who.int/publications/2007/9789241595230_eng.pdf

Hoskin, K. 1996. 'The "Awful Idea of Accountability": Inscribing People into the Measurement of Objects', in Munro, R. and Mouritsen, J. (eds), *Accountaibility: Power, Ethos and the Technologies of Managing.* London: International Thomson Business Press, pp. 265–282.

Howie, P., Forsyth, J., Ogston, S., Clark, A. and Florey, C. 1990. 'Protective Effect of Breastfeeding against Infection', *British Medical Journal* 300: 11–16.

Hume, D. 2000 [1739/40]. 'Treatise on Human Nature', in Norton, D. and Norton, M. (eds), *Treatise on Human Nature.* Oxford: Oxford University Press.

Ip, S., Cheung, M., Raman, G., Chew, P., Magula, N., DeVine, D., Trikalinos, T. and Lau, J. 2007. 'Breastfeeding and Maternal and Infant Health Outcomes in Developed Countries: Evidence Report/ Technology Assessment', Report 153. Rockville, MA: Agency for Healthcare Research and Quality.

Jain, A., Concato, J. and Leventhal, J. 2002. 'How Good Is the Evidence Linking Breastfeeding and Intelligence?' *Pediatrics* 109(6): 1044–1053.

Jenkins, J. and Valiente. M. 1994. 'Bodily Transactions of the Passion: El Calor among Salvadorian Women Refugees', in Csordas, T. (ed.), *Embodiment and Experience: The Existential Ground of Culture and Self.* Cambridge: Cambridge University Press, pp. 163–183.

Jenkins, R. 1996. *Social Identity.* London: Routledge.

Jordanova, L. (ed.). 1986. *Languages of Nature: Critical Essays on Science and Literature.* London: Free Association Books.

Kanter, R. 1972. *Commitment and Community Communes and Utopias in Sociological Perspective.* Cambridge, MA: Harvard University Press.

Kanieski, M. 2010. 'Securing attachment: The shifting medicalisation of attachment and attachment disorders' *Heath, Risk and Society* Special Issue: 'Child-rearing in an Age of Risk.' 12: 4, 335–344.

Kaplan, L. 1978. *Oneness and Separateness: From Infant to Individual.* New York: Touchstone Press.

Keck, M. and Sikkink, K. 1998. *Activists Beyond Borders: Advocacy Networks in World Politics.* London: Cornell University Press.

Kennedy, K. and Visness C. 1992. 'Contraceptive Efficacy of Lactational Amenorrhea', *The Lancet* 339: 227–230.

Kitzinger, J. 1990. 'Strategies of the Early Childbirth Movement: A Case-Study of the National Childbirth Trust', in Garcia, J., Kilpatrick, R. and Richards, M. (eds), *The Politics of Maternity Care: Services for Childbearing Women in Twentieth-Century Britain.* Oxford: Clarendon Press, pp. 92–115.

Klaus, M. and Kennell, J. 1976. *Maternal-Infant Bonding: The Impact of Early Separation or Loss on Family Development.* St. Louis, MO: Mosby.

Klein, G. 1998. *Sources of Power: How People Make Decisions.* Massachusetts: MIT Press.

Klein, M. 1975. *Love Guilt, Reparation, and Other Works 1921–1945.* New York: Delacorte Press.

Kleinman, A. 1995. *Writing at the Margin: Discourse Between Anthropology and Medicine.* Berkeley, Los Angeles and London: University of California Press.

Klement, E., Cohen, R., Bowman, J., Joseph, A. and Reif, S. 2005. 'Breast-feeding and Risk of Inflammatory Bowel Disease: A Systematic Review with Meta-analysis', *American Journal of Clinical Nutrition* 82(2): 485–486.

Knaak, S. 2005. 'Breast-Feeding, Bottle-Feeding and Dr Spock: The Shifting Context of Choice', *Canadian Review of Sociology and Anthropology* 42(2): 197–216.

Knaak, S. 2006. 'The Problem with Breastfeeding Discourse', *Canadian Journal of Public Health* 97(5): 412–414.

Kneidel, S. 1990. 'Nursing Beyond One Year', *New Beginnings* 6(4): 99–103.

Kramer, M. 2001. 'Promotion of Breastfeeding Intervention Trial (PROBIT): A Randomized Trial in the Republic of Belarus', *Journal of the American Medical Association* 285(4): 413–420.

Kukla, R. 2005. *Mass Hysteria: Medicine, Culture and Women's Bodies.* New York: Rowman & Littlefield.

Latour, B. 1993. *We Have Never Been Modern,* trans. Catherine Porter. Cambridge, MA: Harvard University Press.

Latour, B. and Woolgar, S. 1986. *Laboratory Life: The Construction of Scientific Facts.* Princeton, NJ: Princeton University Press.

Lavelli, M. and Polli, M. 1998. 'Early Mother-Infant Interaction During Breast and Bottle Feeding', *Infant Behaviour and Development* 21(4): 667–684.

Law, J. 2000. 'The Politics of Breastfeeding: Assessing Risk, Dividing Labor', *Signs* 25(2): 407–450.

Layne, L. 2006. 'Pregnancy and Infant Loss Support: A New, Feminist, American, Patient Movement?' *Social Science and Medicine* 62: 602–613.

Lee, E. 2007a. 'Health, Morality, and Infant Feeding: British Mothers' Experiences of Formula Milk Use in the Early Weeks', *Sociology of Health and Illness* 29(7): 1075–1090.

Lee, E. 2007b. 'Infant Feeding in Risk Society', *Health, Risk and Society* 9(3): 295–309.

Lee, E. 2008. 'Living with Risk in the Age of "Intensive Motherhood": Maternal Identity and Infant Feeding', *Health, Risk and Society* 10(5): 467–477.

Lee, E. 2011. 'Feeding Babies and the Problem of Policy', CPCS Briefing. Retrieved 31 March 2011 from http://blogs.kent.ac.uk/parentingculturestudies/files/2011/02/CPCS-Briefing-on-feeding-babies-FINAL-revised1.pdf

Lee, E. and Bristow, J. 2009. 'Rules for Feeding Babies', in Day Sclater, S., Ebtehaj, F., Jackson, E. and Richards, M. (eds), *Regulating Autonomy: Sex Reproduction and Family.* Oxford: Hart, pp. 73–91.

Lee, E. Faircloth, C. Macvarish, J and Bristow, J. Forthcoming. *Blame the Parents? A Brief Introduction to Parenting Culture Studies,* Palgrave Macmillan.

Lee, E. and Furedi, F. 2005. 'Mothers' Experience of, and Attitudes to, Using Infant Formula in the Early Months', School of Sociology, Sociology and Social Research: University of Kent at Canterbury. Retrieved 4 September 2006 from http://www.kent.ac.uk/sspssr/staff/academic/lee/infant-formula-summary.pdf

Lee, E., Macvarish, J. and Bristow, J. 2010. 'Editorial: Risk, Health and Parenting Culture', *Health Risk and Society* 12(4): 293–300.

Liedloff, J. 1985. *The Continuum Concept: In Search of Happiness Lost.* Reading, MA: Addison-Wesley.

LLLI (La Leche League International). 1998. 'LLLI Policies and Standing Rules Notebooks, Appendix 1' (rev. Feb 1998), in *La Leche League Purpose and Philosophy.* Schaumberg, IL: LLLI.

LLLI. 2000. 'The LLL Leader and the IBCLC - A Partnership in Breastfeeding History', *Leaven* 36(3): 52–53.

LLLI. 2003. *The Breastfeeding Answer Book,* 3rd rev. ed. Chicago: LLLI.

LLLI. 2004. Bylaws. Retrieved 4 April 2007 from http://www.llli.org/bylaws.html

LLLI. 2004. *The Womanly Art of Breastfeeding.* 7th rev. ed. Chicago: LLLI.

LLLI. 2008. Annual Review. Retrieved 13 April 2011 from http://www.laleche.org.uk/pdfs/AnnualReview2008(final).pdf

LLLFrance. 2006. National Congress. October 29th 2006, Paris.

LLLGB. 2008. Peer Counsellor Programme. Retrieved 17 December 2008 from http://www.lllgbpcp.org.uk/ now http://www.laleche.org.uk/pages/about/pcp_about.htm

Loizos, P. and Heady, P. 1999. *Conceiving Persons: Ethnographies of Procreation, Fertility and Growth,* London School of Economics Monographs on Social Anthropology 68. London: Athlone Press.

Lorenz, K. 1937. 'The Nature of Instinct', in Schiller, C. (ed.), *Instinctive Behavior: The Development of a Modern Concept.* London: Methuen, pp. 129–175.

Lorenz, K. 1950. 'The Comparative Method of Studying Innate Behavior Patterns', *Symposia for the Society of Experimental Biology* 4: 221–268.

Lucas, A., Morley, R., Cole, T. and Gore, S. 1994. 'A Randomized Multicenter Study of Human Milk versus Formula and Later Development in Preterm Infants', *Archives of Disease in Childhood* 70: F141.46.

Lupton, D. 1996. *Food, the Body and the Self.* London: Sage.

Maher, J. and Saugeres, L. 2007. 'To Be or Not to Be a Mother? Women Negotiating Cultural Representations of Mothering', *Journal of Sociology* 43(1): 5–21.

Maher, V. 1992. *The Anthropology of Breastfeeding: Natural Law or Social Construct?* Oxford: Berg.

Mainstream Parenting Resources. 2008. 'Following Your Instincts, Part I.' Retrieved 4 February 2009 from http://mainstreamparenting.wordpress .com/2008/01/04/following-your-instincts-part-i/

Marild, S., Jodal, U. and Hanson, L. 1990. 'Breastfeeding and Urinary Tract Infection' [letter], *The Lancet* 336: 942.

Marini, A., Agosti, M., Motta, G. and Misca, F. 1996. 'Effects of a Dietary and Environmental Prevention Programme on the Incidence of Allergic Symptoms in High Atopic Risk Infants: Three Years Follow-up', *Acta Paediatrica Supplement* 414: 1–22.

Marshall, J.L., Godfrey, M. and Renfrew, M.J. 2007. 'Being a "Good Mother": Managing Breastfeeding and Merging Identities', *Social Science and Medicine* 65(10): 2147–2159.

Martin, E. 1987. *The Woman in the Body: A Cultural Analysis of Reproduction.* Boston: Beacon Press.

Martin, E. 1998. 'The Fetus as Intruder: Mothers' Bodies and Medical Metaphors', in Davis-Floyd, R. and Dumit, J. (eds), *Cyborg Babies: From Technosex to Techno-Tots.* New York: Routledge, pp. 125–142.

Marx, K. 1977 [1859]. *A Contribution to the Critique of Political Economy.* Moscow: Progress Publishers.

Massumi, B. 2002a. 'Navigating Movements: A Conversation with Brian Massumi', in Zournazi, M. (ed.), *Hope: New Philosophies for Change.* London: Routledge, pp. 210–243.

Massumi, B. 2002b. *Parables for the Virtual: Movement, Affect, Sensation.* Durham, NC: Duke University Press.

Mauss, M. 1973. 'Techniques of the Body', *Economy and Society* 2(1): 70–88.

McCaughey, M. 2008. *The Caveman Mystique: Pop-Darwinism and the Debates over Sex, Violence and Science.* London: Routledge.

McDonald, M. and Lambert, H. 2009. 'Introduction', in McDonald, M. and Lambert, H. (eds), *Social Bodies.* Oxford: Berghahn Books, pp. 1–17.

McEwen, B. 2000. 'The Neurobiology of Stress: From Serendipity to Clinical Relevance', *Brain Research* 886: 172–189.

McNamara, D. 2006. 'Parental Control, Overprotection Associated with Anxiety in Children', *Clinical Psychiatry News* 34(1): 44.

Mead, G.H. 1934. *Mind, Self, and Society.* Chicago: University of Chicago Press.

Mead, M. 1962. 'A Cultural Anthropologist's Approach to Maternal Deprivation', in Ainsworth, M., Andry, R., Harlow, R., Lebovici, S., Mead, M., Prugh, D. and Wotton, B. (eds), *Deprivation of Maternal Care: A Reassessment of Its Effects.* Geneva: WHO, pp. 45–62.

Menstuff. 2011. Male Lactation. Retrieved 01 April 2011 from http://www .menstuff.org/issues/byissue/malelactation.html

Milkie, M., Mattingly, M., Nomaguchi, K., Bianchi, S. and Robinson, J. 2004. 'The Time Squeeze: Parental Statuses and Feelings about Time with Children', *Journal of Marriage and Family* 66(3): 739–761.

Miller, D. 1997. 'How Infants Grow Mothers in North London', *Theory, Culture and Society* 14: 67–88.

Miller, T. 2005. *Making Sense of Motherhood: A Narrative Approach*. Cambridge: Cambridge University Press.

Miller, T., Bonas, S. and Dixon-Woods, M. 2007. 'Qualitative Research on Breastfeeding in the UK: A Narrative Review and Methodological Reflection', *Evidence and Policy* 3(2): 197–230.

Mortensen, E., Michaelsen, K., Sanders, S. and Reinisch, J. 2002. 'The Association between Duration of Breastfeeding and Adult Intelligence', *Journal of the American Medical Association* 28(15): 2365–2371.

Moscucci, O. 2003. 'Holistic Obstetrics: The Origins of "Natural Childbirth" in Britain', *Postgraduate Medical Journal* 79: 168–173.

Mosse, D. 2006. 'Anti-Social Anthropology? Objectivity, Objection, and the Ethnography of Public Policy and Professional Communities', *Journal of the Royal Anthropological Institute* 12(4): 935–956.

MS (Ministère des Solidarités, de la Santé et de la Famille). 2005. 'Allaitement Maternel : Les Bénéfices pour la Santé de l'Enfant et de sa Mere. Les Synthèses du Programme National Nutrition-santé'. Retrieved 23 April 2009 from www.sante.gouv.fr/htm/pointsur/nutrition/allaitement.pdf)

Munro, R. and Mouritsen, J. (eds). 1996. *Accountability: Power, Ethos and the Technologies of Managing*. London: International Thomson Business Press.

Murphy, E. 1999. '"Breast Is Best": Infant Feeding Decisions and Maternal Deviance', *Sociology of Health and Illness* 21(2): 187–208.

Murphy, E. 2003. 'Expertise and Forms of Knowledge in the Government of Families', *Sociological Review* 51(4): 433–462.

National Statistics Online 2008. 'Births and Patterns of Family Building: England and Wales'. Retrieved 12 August 2008 from http://www.statistics.gov.uk/statbase/Product.asp?vlnk=5768

Newman, J. 1995. 'How Breastmilk Protects Newborns', *Scientific American* 273(6): 76–79.

NHS. 2009. NHS Pregnancy Planner. Retrieved 25 February 2009 from http://www.nhs.uk/planners/pregnancycareplanner/pages/birthplan.aspx

Oddy, W., Holt, P., Sly, P., Peat, J. and de Klerk, N. 2002. 'Maternal Asthma, Infant Feeding, and the Risk of Asthma in Childhood', *Journal of Allergy and Clinical Immunology* 110: 65–67.

OECD. 2009. LFS by Sex and Age. Retrieved 26 February 2009 from http://stats.oecd.org/Index.aspx?DatasetCode=LFS_D

Pain, R., Bailey, C. and Mowl G. 2001. 'Infant Feeding in North East England: Contested Spaces of Reproduction', *Area* 33(3): 261–272.

Palmer, G. 1993 [1988]. *The Politics of Breastfeeding*, 2nd ed. London: Pandora Press.

Perry, B., Pollard, R., Blakeley, T., Baker, W. and Vigilante, D. 1995. 'Childhood Trauma, the Neurobiology of Adaptation and 'Use-Dependent' Development of the Brain: How "States" Become "Traits"', *Infant Mental Health Journal* 16: 271–291.

Persson et al. 1998. 'The Helen Keller International Food-Frequency Method Underestimates Vitamin A Intake Where Sustained Breastfeeding Is Common', *Food and Nutrition Bulletin* 19(4) Retrieved 1 October 2007 from http://www.unu.edu/unupress/food/fub19-4.pdf now http://global-breastfeeding.org/pdf/persson_BM.pdf

Petchesky, R. 1987. 'Foetal Images: The Power of Visual Culture in the Politics of Reproduction', in Stanworth, M. (ed.), *Reproductive Technologies: Gender, Motherhood and Medicine*. Oxford: Polity, pp. 57–80.

Peterson, A. and Lupton, D. 1996. *The New Public Health: Health and Self in the Age of Risk*. London: Sage.

Phoenix, A. Wollett, A. and Lloyd, E. (eds). 1991. *Motherhood: Meanings, Practices and Ideologies*. London: Sage.

Piaget, J. 1955. *The Child's Construction of Reality*. London: Routledge and Kegan Paul.

Piper, H. and Sikes, P. 2010. 'Researching Barriers to Cultural Change for Those in Loco Parentis', *Sociological Research Online* (Special Section 'Changing Parenting Culture') 15(4). Retrieved 1 June 2011 from http://www.socresonline.org.uk/15/4/5.html

Pishva, N., Mehryar, M., Mahmoudi, H. and Farzan, R. 1998. 'Application of Topical Breast Milk for Prevention of Neonatal Conjunctivitis', *Journal of Medical Science* 23 (1–2): 55.

Porter, L. 2008. 'The Science of Attachment: The Biological Roots of Love.' Issue 119, July/August 2003. Retrieved 8 March 2008 from http://www.mothering.com/community/a/the-science-of-attachment-the-biological-roots-of-love

Power, M. 1994. *The Audit Explosion*. London: Demos.

Prescott, J. 1997. 'Breastfeeding: Brain Nutrients in Brain Development for Human Love and Peace', *Touch The Future Newsletter* (Spring). Retrieved 5 June 2008 from http://www.violence.de/prescott/ttf/article.html

Pugh, A. 2005. 'Selling Compromise: Toys, Motherhood, and the Cultural Deal', *Gender and Society* 19: 729–749.

Radcliffe-Brown, A. 1952. *Structure and Function in Primitive Society*. London: Cohen and West.

Ragoné, H. 1994. *Surrogate Motherhood: Conception in the Heart*. Oxford: Westview Press.

Ramaekers, S. and Suissa, J. 2011. *The Claims of Parenting: Reasons, Responsibility and Society*, Contemporary Philosophies and Theories in Education 4. London: Springer.

Raphael, D. and Davis, F. 1985. *Only Mothers Know: Patterns of Infant Feeding in Traditional Cultures*. Westport, CT, and London: Greenwood Press (published by the Human Lactation Center Ltd).

Rapley, G. 2006. 'Baby-Led Weaning', in Dykes, F. and Hall Moran, V. (eds), *Maternal and Infant Nutrition and Nurture: Controversies and Challenges*. London: Quay Books, pp. 275–299.

Rapp, R. 2000. *Testing Women, Testing the Fetus: The Social Impact of Amniocentesis in America*. London and New York: Routledge.

Reeve, J. 1997. 'Message in a Bottle: A Dissertation that Addresses the Question "What Messages do Health Professionals Give to Mothers on the Subject of Infant Feeding?"' Ph.D. dissertation. Department of Social Anthropology, University of Cambridge.

Renfrew, M., et al. 2005. *The Effectiveness of Public Health Interventions to Promote the Duration of Breastfeeding: A Systematic Review.* London: National Institute for Clinical Excellence.

Riggs, J. 2005. 'Impressions of Mothers and Fathers on the Periphery of Child Care', *Psychology of Women Quarterly* 29: 58–62.

Robinson, V. 2007. *The Drinks Are On Me: Everything Your Mother Never Told You About Breastfeeding.* East Grinstead: Art of Change Press.

Rogan, W. and Gladen, B. 1993. 'Breastfeeding and Cognitive Development', *Early Human Development* 31: 181–193.

Rogers, I., Emmett, P. and Golding, J. 1997. 'The Incidence and Duration of Breast Feeding', *Early Human Development* 49: S45–S74. doi:10.1016/S0378-3782(97)00053-4.

Rose, N. 1999 [1989]. *Governing the Soul: The Shaping of the Private Self.* London: Routledge.

Rose, N. and Novas, C. 2004. 'Biological Citizenship', in Ong, A. and Collier, S. (eds), *Global Assemblages: Technology, Politics, and Ethics as Anthropological Problems.* Oxford: Blackwell, pp. 439–463.

Rosenblatt, K., Thomas, D. and the WHO Collaborative Study of Neoplasia and Steroid Contraception. 1993. 'Lactation and the Risk of Epithelial Ovarian Cancer', *International Journal of Epidemiology* 22(2): 192–197.

Sachs, M. 2006. 'Routine Weighing of Babies: Does It Improve Feeding and Care?' *Journal of Child Health Care* 10: 90–95.

Sadauskaite-Kuehne, V., Ludvigsson, J., Padaiga, Z., Jasinskiene, E. and Samuelsson, U. 2004. 'Longer Breastfeeding Is an Important Protective Factor against Development of Type 1 Diabetes Mellitus in Childhood', *Diabetes/Metabolism Research and Reviews* 20(2): 150–157.

Schiebinger, L. 1993. *Nature's Body: Gender in the Making of Modern Science.* Boston: Beacon Press.

Schmeid, V., Sheehan, A. and Barclay, L. 2001. 'Contemporary Breast-feeding Policy and Practice: Implications for Midwives', *Midwifery* 17: 44–54.

Schmidt, J. 2008. 'Gendering in Infant Feeding Discourses: The Good Mother and the Absent Father', *New Zealand Sociology* 23(2): 61–74.

Schneider, D. 1969. 'Kinship, Nationality and Religion in American Culture: Towards a Definition of Kinship', in Spencer, R. (ed.), *Forms of Symbolic Action: Proceedings of the 1969 Annual Spring Meeting of the American Ethnological Society.* Seattle: University of Washington Press, pp. 116–125.

Schore, A. 2001. 'The Effects of Early Relational Trauma on Right Brain Development, Affect Regulation and Infant Mental Health', *Infant Mental Health Journal* 22(1–2): 201–269.

Scott, J. 1995. *Weapons of the Weak: Everyday Forms of Peasant Resistance.* London: Yale University Press.

Scott, J. 2003. 'Women's Experiences of Breastfeeding in a Bottle-Feeding Culture', *Journal of Human Lactation* 19(3): 270–277.

Sears, W. 2003. *Becoming a Father.* Schaumberg, IL: LLLI.

Sears, W. and Sears, M. 1993 [1982]. *The Baby Book: Everything You Need to Know About Your Baby*. Boston: Little Brown.

Sears, W. and Sears, M. 2001. *The Attachment Parenting Book: A Commonsense Guide to Understanding and Nurturing Your Baby*. London: Little, Brown and Company.

Shah, P., Aliwalas, L. and Shah, V. 2006. 'Breastfeeding or Breast Milk to Alleviate Procedural Pain in Neonates: A Systematic Review', *Cochrane Database Systematic Review* 3: CD004950.

Shaw, R. 2003. 'Theorizing Breastfeeding: Body Ethics, Maternal Generosity and the Gift Relation', *Body and Society* 9(2): 55–73.

Shaw, S. 2008. 'Family Leisure and Changing Ideologies of Parenthood', *Sociology Compass* 2: 688–703.

Shostak, M. 1981. *Nisa: the Life and Words of a !Kung Woman*. New York: Random House.

Shostak, M. 2000. *Return to Nisa*. Cambridge, MA: Harvard University Press.

Sinnott, A. 2010. *Breastfeeding Older Children*. London: Free Association Books.

Slade, H. and Schwartz, S. 1987. 'Mucosal Immunity: The Immunology of Breast Milk', *Journal of Allergy and Clinical Immunology* 80(3, part 1): 348–358.

Small, M. 1998. *Our Babies, Ourselves: How Biology and Culture Shape the Way We Parent*. New York: Random House.

Spangler, G., Schieche, M., Ilg, U., Maier, U. and Ackerman, C. 1994. 'Maternal Sensitivity as an Organizer for Biobehavioral Regulation in Infancy', *Developmental Psychobiology* 27: 425–437.

Stapleton, H., Fielder, A. and Kirkham, M. 2008. 'Breast or Bottle? Eating Disordered Childbearing Women and Infant-Feeding Decisions', *Maternal and Child Nutrition* 4(2): 106–120.

Strathern, M. 1981. *Kinship at the Core: An Anthropology of Elmdon, A Village in North-West Essex in the Nineteen-Sixties*. Cambridge: Cambridge University Press.

Strathern, M. 1982. 'No Nature, No Culture: The Hagan Case', in MacCormack, C. and Strathern, M. (eds), *Nature, Culture and Gender*. Cambridge, Cambridge University Press, pp. 174–223.

Strathern, M. 1987. 'The Limits of Auto-anthropology', in Jackson, A. (ed.), *Anthropology at Home*, ASA Monographs 25. London and New York: Tavistock Publications, pp. 16–37.

Strathern, M. 1992a. 'Parts and Wholes: Refiguring Relationships in a Postplural World', in Kuper, A. (ed.), *Conceptualising Society*. London: Routledge, pp. 25–103.

Strathern, M. 1992b. *After Nature: Kinship in the Late Twentieth Century*. Cambridge: Cambridge University Press.

Strathern, M. 1993. *Reproducing the Future: Anthropology, Kinship and the New Reproductive Technologies*. Manchester: Manchester University Press.

Strathern, M. 1997. 'From Improvement to Enhancement: An Anthropological Comment on the Audit Culture', *Cambridge Anthropology* 19: 1–21.

Strathern, M. 2005. *Kinship, Law and the Unexpected: Relatives Are Always a Surprise.* Cambridge: Cambridge University Press.

Strathern, M. (ed.). 2000. *Audit Cultures: Anthropological Studies in Accountability, Ethics and the Academy.* London: Routledge.

Stryker, S. 1968. 'Identity Salience and Role Performance: The Importance of Symbolic Interaction Theory for Family Research', *Journal of Marriage and the Family* 30: 558–564.

Suizzo, M.-A. 2004. 'Mother-Child Relationships in France: Balancing Autonomy and Affiliation in Everyday Interactions', *Ethos* 32: 293–323.

Sunderland, M. 2006. *The Science of Parenting: Practical Guidance on Sleep, Crying, Play and Building Emotional Wellbeing for Life.* London: Dorling Kindersley.

Sutherland, K. 1999. 'Of Milk and Miracles: Nursing, the Life Drive, and Subjectivity', *Frontiers: A Journal of Women Studies* 20(2) ('Motherhood and Maternalism'): 1–20.

Taren, D. and Chen, J. 'A Positive Association between Extended Breastfeeding and Nutritional Status in Rural Hubei Province, People's Republic of China', *American Journal of Clinical Nutrition* 58: 862–867.

Textor, J. 1967. *A Cross Cultural Summary.* New Haven, CT: HRAF Press.

The Breastmilk Baby. 2011. Retrieved 31 March 2011 from http://thebreast milkbaby.com/

Thomas, P. 2006. 'Suck On This', *The Ecologist* (April). Retrieved 9 June 2009 from http://www.theecologist.org/pages/archive_detail.asp?content_id= 586 now http://www.theecologist.org/investigations/health/268712/suck _on_this.html

Tiefer, L. 2004. *Sex Is Not a Natural Act and Other Essays.* Boulder, CO: Westview Press.

Tomori, C. 2010. 'Managing Nighttime Breastfeeding in Parenting: Negotiating Personhood, Kinship and Capitalism', *American Anthropological Association Meetings,* 17–21 November 2010 New Orleans.

Trivers, R. 1974. 'Parent-Offspring Conflict', *American Zoologist* 14(1): 249–264.

Tronick, E. and Weinberg, M. 1997. 'Depressed Mothers and Infants: Failure to Form Dyadic States of Consciousness', in Murray, L. and Cooper, P. (eds), *Postpartum Depression in Child Development.* New York: Guilford Press, pp. 54–84.

Tronto, J.C. 2002. 'The "Nanny" Question in Feminism', *Hypatia* 17: 34–51.

Umansky, L. 1998. 'Breastfeeding in the 1990s: The Karen Carter Case and the Politics of Maternal Sexuality', in Umansky, L. and Ladd-Taylor, M., (eds) *'Bad Mothers': The Politics of Blame in Twentieth-Century America.* New York: New York University Press, pp. 299–310.

UNICEF. 2005. The Baby Friendly Initiative. Retrieved 3 December 2006 from http://www.babyfriendly.co.uk now http://www.unicef.org.uk/ babyfriendly/

UNICEF, The National Childbirth Trust and Save the Children. 2007. *A Weak Formula for Legislation: How Loopholes in the Law are Putting Babies at Risk.*

London: UNICEF. Retrieved 4 December 2010 from http://www.unicef
.org.uk/Documents/Baby_Friendly/Statements/feedingreport.pdf

United Kingdom National Case-Control Study Group. 1993. 'Breastfeeding
and the Risk of Breast Cancer in Young Women', *British Medical Journal*
307: 17–20.

Van Esterick, P. 1989. *Beyond the Breast-Bottle Controversy.* New Brunswick,
NJ: Rutgers University Press.

van Ijzendoorn, M. and Kroonberg, P. 1988. 'Cross-Cultural Patterns of Attachment: A Meta-Analysis of the Strange Situation', *Child Development*
59: 147–156.

Victoria, C., Vaughan, J., Lombardi, C., Fuchs, S., Gigante, L., Smith, P.,
Noble, L., Texeira, A., Moreira, L. and Barros, F. 1987. 'Evidence for Pro-
tection by Breastfeeding against Infant Death from Infectious Diseases in
Brazil', *The Lancet* 7: 319–322.

Wagner, R. 1981 [1975]. *The Invention of Culture.* London: University of Chicago Press.

Wall, G. 2001. 'Moral Constructions of Motherhood in Breastfeeding Discourse', *Gender and Society* 15(4): 592–610.

Wall, G. and Arnold, S. 2007. 'How Involved Is Involved Fathering?' *Gender
and Society* 21(4): 508–527.

Ward, J. 2000. *La Leche League: At the Crossroads of Medicine, Feminism, and Religion.* Chapel Hill and London: University of North Carolina Press.

Warner, J. 2006. *Perfect Madness: Motherhood in the Age of Anxiety.* London:
Vermilion.

Weiner, L. 1994. 'Reconstructing Motherhood: The La Leche League in
Postwar America', *Journal of American History* 80(4): 1357–1381.

Wells, J. 2006. 'The Role of Cultural Factors in Human Breastfeeding: Adaptive Behaviour or Biopower?' in Bose, K. (ed.), *Ecology, Culture, Nutrition,
Health and Disease.* Delhi: Kamla-Raj Enterprises pp. 39–47.

WHO (World Health Organization). 2003. *Global Strategy on Infant and Young
Child Feeding.* Geneva: WHO. Retrieved 27 September 2007 from http://
www.who.int/child-adolescenthealth/New_Publications/NUTRITION/
gs_iycf.pdf now http://www.who.int/nutrition/topics/global_strategy/
en/index.html

Wilkinson, P. 1971. *Social Movement.* London: Pall Mall Press.

Williams, R. 1988 [1976]. *Keywords: A Vocabulary of Culture and Society.* London: Fontana.

Willmott, H. 1996. 'Thinking Accountability: Accounting for the Disciplined
Production of Self', in Munro, R. and Mouritsen, J. (eds), *Accountabil-
ity: Power, Ethos and the Technologies of Managing.* International Thompson
Business Press, pp. 23–39.

Wilson, A. 1980. 'The Infancy of the History of Childhood: An Appraisal of
Philippe Ariès', *History and Theory* 19(2): 132–153.

Wolf, Jacqueline. 2001. *Don't Kill Your Baby: Public Health and the Decline of
Breastfeeding in the 19th and 20th Centuries.* Columbus: Ohio State University Press.

Wolf, Joan. 2011. *Is Breast Best? Taking on the Breastfeeding Experts and the New High Stakes of Motherhood.* New York and London: New York University Press.

Wolf, Naomi. 2001. *Misconceptions: Truth, Lies and the Unexpected on the Journey to Motherhood.* London: Chatto and Windus.

Wolfenstein, M. 1955. 'French Parents Take their Children to the Park', in Mead, M. and Wolfenstein, M. (eds), *Childhood in Contemporary Cultures.* London: University of Chicago Press, pp. 99–117.

Woodburn, J. 2006. 'Extended Breastfeeding', *Salon Magazine.* Retrieved 28 August 2006 from http://www.salon.com/2006/09/18/extended_breastfeeding/

Zelizer, V. 1985. *Pricing the Priceless Child: The Changing Social Value of Children.* Princeton, NJ: Princeton University Press.

INDEX